Managing Cog........ ......

in Parkinson's & Lewy Body Dementia

Helen Buell Whitworth, MS, BSN

James A. Whitworth,
Lewy Body Dementia Association Co-founder

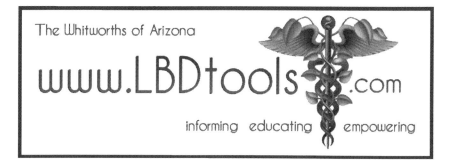

The Whitworths of Arizona

www.LBDtools.com

informing educating empowering

Cover design: Sue Smith and Helen Buell Whitworth

Editors: Leanne Schroyer and Sharon Daniels

The information and opinions herein should be considered an educational service only, designed to provide helpful information. It is not intended to replace a physician's judgment about a diagnosis, treatment, or therapy. Readers who fail to consult appropriate health authorities must assume the risk of any injuries. The authors and publisher disclaim any responsibility and liability of any kind in connection with the reader's use of the information contained herein. References are provided for informational purposes only and do not constitute endorsement of any websites or other sources. Readers should be aware that the websites listed in this book may change.

Copyright © 2015 The Whitworths of Arizona

All rights reserved.

ISBN-10: 1-5146712-2-0

ISBN-13: 978-1-514671-2-21

Other books by the Whitworths

A Caregiver's Guide to Lewy Body Dementia (2010). A thorough overview of Lewy body dementia and how to deal with it. *"This book is the most helpful book I have read about Lewy body dementia! It is like a field guide for caring for someone with Lewy Body!"* One of the many five-star reviews on Amazon.

Riding a Rollercoaster with Lewy Body Dementia (2009). A textbook for staff. Presently only available as a textbook for care staff. *"It was easy to understand but thorough. I learned so much."* Review from a registered nurse.

Books by Helen Buell Whitworth

On the Road with the Whitworths: A Thrifty Couple's Tribulations and Triumphs (2015). Get to know the Whitworths as you read about the start of their work with LBD and their first summer of RVing in Rex, their "new" secondhand motor home. *"I loved it. It was hilarious."* Reader's review.

Betsy (Second edition, 2014, First edition, 2006) A romantic novel based on Helen's family history. Fiction written in the same relaxed manner as the above books. *"An enjoyable read. I couldn't put it down until I was done."* Reader's review.

All books are available on LBDtools.com.

Dedication

This book is dedicated to the many Parkinson's families we met while writing this book. Their hopes and fears guided much of our writing. We hope that this book can increase their quality of life and decrease their fears.

This book is also dedicated to the many Lewy body dementia support groups that we have visited over the years. They have provided us with great insight into the life of the Lewy team, with their stories, questions, worries and joys.

Acknowledgments

We would like to thank the many people who helped us to make this book possible. Our wonderful writing group, the Red Mountain Writers, helped us to keep our book easy to read, always our aim. Our readers, Ali Koman, Marla Burns and Leanne Schroyer all had good input. The book would not have been the same without them. Pat Snyder has been especially helpful, providing great insight and allowing us to quote from her own book, *Treasures in the Darkness*, at will. Dr. James Leverenz was gracious enough to review our book and write the forward, as well as adding his own guidance in many places, based on his many years of working with this population. Dr. Geri Hall, who has worked with dementia caregivers for many years, also took the time to review our book and provide valuable direction. And finally, Regina Hucks provided great publishing contacts and guidance.

Contents

Forward by James Leverenz, M.D.

I was quite pleased when the Whitworths asked me to write the foreword to their book, *Managing Cognitive Issues in Parkinson's & Lewy Body Dementia*. I have known the authors for some time and have always appreciated their knowledge and insights. I often recommend their previous book, *Caregivers Guide to Lewy Body Dementia* to my patients and their families.

I first met Jim and Helen during the early days of the Lewy Body Dementia Association (LBDA) and have worked with them on several educational projects--we've made a good tag team. As a physician with over 20 years of treating and studying the Lewy body dementias and the chair of the Scientific Advisory Council for the LBDA for four years, I have always found their insights to be illuminating. Thus, I looked forward to gaining new insights on the Lewy body disorders from their new book.

With much that a family and caregiver might want to know about the Lewy body disorders, it didn't disappoint me. Because of their long personal and professional experience with the Lewy body disorders they provide not only the "facts", but also real life examples. The stories and quotes are only too familiar for those of us who deal with these devastating diseases.

The book begins with an overview of some of the medical aspects of these disorders. It goes on to cover the major components including both the motor problems and the non-motor issues such as changes in thinking skills or behaviors.

Understanding the unique aspects of these diseases can be particularly valuable to the caregivers, including the occasional need to educate their loved one's own medical professionals. This is definitely a group of diseases where it is helpful, and sometimes essential, for the caregivers to be advocates and educators. For those who want more "biology", the Whitworths have even added in some pathology and biochemistry.

After this impressive medical overview, the book covers the equally important non-medical aspects. Again, using telling examples they allow the reader to understand the impact of the disease on the caregiver, family, and person suffering with the disease. They offer up important approaches to confronting the disease and the wide variety of therapies that are available.

As a physician that works in this field, I am often frustrated by comments that "there is nothing that you can do". That couldn't be further from the truth and the Whitworths give you the tools to help manage the disease and its effects on the person suffering with it and those around that person.

Many diseases are not cured (e.g., hypertension, diabetes, heart disease), but management can truly improve the quality of life for everyone affected by the disease. Admittedly, when the disease affects one's motor function, thinking skills, and behavior, the challenges can be great. However, there are ways to help everyone through the process. The Whitworths do an admirable job in outlining how this can be done.

The Lewy body diseases are likely the second or third most common cause of dementia (loss of thinking skills and ability to manage day to day functions) in this country, and probably the world. As the world ages, the number of people suffering from the Lewy body diseases and other causes of dementia will double and even triple as we move toward the middle of this century.

We need help to deal with this epidemic. Physicians and researchers must continue to push forward with research to find better ways to treat these diseases and ultimately to cure or prevent their onset. We also need the community engaged in this fight and, thankfully, the Whitworths have committed to this fight.

James B. Leverenz, MD

Director, Cleveland Lou Ruvo Center for Brain Health

Dr. Joseph Hahn Chair of the Neurological Institute, Cleveland Clinic

Chair, Scientific Advisory Council, Lewy Body Dementia Association

Semantics and Acronyms

Most writers put their glossary at the back. However, we want our readers to understand up front what they are reading. Here are some terms and acronyms used regularly. You will find other definitions in handy to find boxes spread throughout the book.

Terms:

Dementia: A group of symptoms pertaining to the loss of cognitive skills such as memory, thinking, or impulse control, severe enough to interfere with functional ability or activities of daily living. Many causes including LBD, Alzheimer's disease, stroke, and others.

Disorder: A group of symptoms pertaining to a variety of issues, which can include cognition, with a common probable cause and outcome.

Lewy body disorder: A disorder at least partially caused by Lewy bodies.

Lewy body dementia (LBD): An umbrella term for two sister dementias: Parkinson's disease with dementia (PDD) and dementia with Lewy bodies (DLB). In this book, the term Lewy body dementia or LBD is used unless the information is specific to either PDD or DLB.

He and she: Because there are more men with Lewy body disorders than women,[1] the authors occasionally use a generic "he" for PwLB and an equally generic "she" for care partners. This does not discount the many women with Lewy body disorders, like co-author James Whitworth's own Annie, or male care partners like James. It simply makes for an easier read.

Lewy team: The person at risk for a Lewy body disorder and the primary care partner. Most often called "caregiver and loved one" we have usually chosen to use this more inclusive term.

Care partner vs. caregiver: Parkinson's teams usually refer to care partners, while LBD teams usually refer to caregivers. As the job changes, so does the title.

Lewy-sensitive drug: One where a normal dose may act as an overdose or have an adverse (opposite) reaction with LBD. These drugs will vary with each patient although certain drug families are more likely to be Lewy sensitive than others.

Pre-dementia disorders: Those Lewy body disorders that can occur prior to dementia: REM sleep behavior disorder, Parkinsons disease and mild cognitive impairment of the Lewy body type.

Mild cognitive impairment, Lewy body type. Non-amnestic mild cognitive impairment, where thinking skills are impaired more than memory, but are still mild enough that they do not interfere with day to day functioning. This is the type that usually precedes Lewy body dementia.

Acronyms

LB: Lewy bodies.

LBD: Lewy body disorder/dementia, an umbrella term for the following two disorders:

PDD: Parkinson's disease with dementia, the type of Lewy body dementia that starts after a PD diagnosis.

DLB: Dementia with Lewy bodies, the type of Lewy body disorder that starts with dementia.

PD: Parkinson's disease, a Lewy body disorder that affects mobility.

RBD: REM sleep behavior disorder, sometimes called "Active Dreams," a Lewy body disorder which often precedes Parkinson's disease and Lewy body dementia.

MCI-LB: Mild cognitive impairment-Lewy body type, (or non-amnestic MCI) Usually shortened to "MCI" in this book, it will be called "amnestic MCI or MCI-AD" when the type that usually precedes Alzheimer's is meant.

Pw(disorder acronym): Designates the person/people with (disorder).

PwPD means person/people with Parkinson's disease.

PwLB means person/people with a Lewy body disorder, usually where the dementia status is unknown, absent or very mild.

PwLBD means person/people with Lewy body dementia.

PwAD means person/people with Alzheimer's disease.

Introduction

The goal of this book is to provide support to people with Parkinson's disease (PD) and others at risk for Lewy body dementia (LBD) through better knowledge of the disorder and its symptoms. While people tend to shy away from the thought of cognitive degeneration, it is not rare with PD and can even occur before motor symptoms.

When a family learns about the possibility of dementia, they may feel as though they are on a runaway train rushing towards a fearful and uncontrollable future. This book offers knowledge and methods of control to replace that fear and helplessness.

It is true that no one has found a way to cure dementia. According to Dr. James Galvin, neurologist at Florida Atlantic University in Boca Raton, FL, "The most that [drugs] have been able to do so far is slow down the symptoms' progress without changing the underlying disease. There's no way to repair the damage that's been done."[2]

Like drugs, living a healthy lifestyle, stress management, or any other alternative therapy will not cure dementia or stop its progress. However, we believe that many ways are safer than drugs, and often as effective, for slowing symptom progress, decreasing symptom severity and thus, increasing quality of life.

While it is well known that many drugs can react poorly with Lewy body disorders, not all drugs are bad. Some can be very helpful. The authors—and a growing number of physicians—

advocate a combination of traditional medicine and alternative therapies to provide families with the best of both modalities.

The earlier the possibility of LBD is identified, the more you can do to ease the journey. Throughout this book, symptoms will be mentioned as often being the first symptom noticed, especially on retrospect. That's because people with Lewy body disorders vary greatly as to what symptoms they have at all and what ones show up first. Any of the symptoms mentioned could be the ones YOU notice first. Knowing what they are and being observant will help you to identify the possibility of dementia early enough to keep the symptoms milder and less troublesome for a longer time.

Lewy body disorders are progressively degenerative; no one can get off the train—not yet anyway. However, you can do a lot to keep the symptoms milder for a longer period of time and make the journey smoother.

This book is for anyone dealing with:

- Parkinson's disease (PD), mild cognitive impairment or any other disorder identified within as risk factors for Lewy body dementia (LBD).
- Unexplained character changes.
- Hallucinations (especially visual), fluency problems, sleep disturbances or other possible early LBD symptoms.
- Lewy body dementia already diagnosed or suspected.

Our Focus

This book is written from the viewpoint of the educated caregiver, rather than a professional. While the opinions the authors share are our own, they are voiced by other caregivers as well. We draw heavily on Helen's background of psychology and nursing and James's personal experiences with his first wife, many support groups and the Lewy Body Dementia Association. We've supported our work with references to scientific articles, but our books should never be utilized in the place of a qualified physician.

A Caregiver's Guide to Lewy Body Dementia, (the *Guide*), also by the Whitworths, is an excellent reference book. Because it covers important subjects touched upon only lightly here, referrals to the *Guide*, with page numbers, are included when appropriate.

The Lewy Team

The person with or at risk for LBD and the caregiver are a team. While only one has the symptoms, both are affected. Married couple, parent and adult child, siblings, or other caregiver arrangement, the pair are partners in this endeavor.

In the early stages of the disorder, a person with a Lewy body disorder (PwLB) is still in charge, making personal decisions and acting upon them. Even so, this book is written to the care partner. Family members continually report that even PwLB who are still able to read well are seldom interested in reading about their disorder. Most prefer to let their care partners do the research. Thus, it will usually be up to the care partner to read, sift and share the information in this book as the PwLB can tolerate or wishes to hear.

In many ways, this is a very positive book, with a hopeful message. It doesn't promise a cure, but the information here can help to decrease stress, add to your team's quality of life and extend the time before dementia takes over.

The Lewy Body Family of Disorders and Ages When They Tend to Occur

Progression to Parkinson's Disease with Dementia

Age:	20s	30s	40s	50s	60s	70s	80+
RBD:							
MCI-LB:							
PD:							
PDD, a type of LBD:							

Progression to Dementia with Lewy Bodies

Age:	20s	30s	40s	50s	60s	70s	80+
RBD:							
MCI-LB:							
DLB, a type of LBD:							

The darker the line, the more likely the occurrence.

These approximate timelines show the relationship between members of the Lewy body family. A person can have any or all of these disorders but if Parkinson's motor symptoms appear before the dementia, then the progress will be to PDD, not DLB.[3]

Section One:

Learning about Lewy Disorders

For the person with Parkinson's, dementia may not happen at all. If it does, it will not be something that happens overnight. It sneaks up, but it does leave tracks. As conditions such as mild cognitive impairment appear, they warn of possible eventual dementia. The more risk factors, the stronger the possibility. When symptoms such as hallucinations emerge, the likelihood of eventual Lewy body dementia (LBD) becomes more certain.

Knowledge is essential when dealing with this confusing disorder. Because LBD is a comparatively new disease, doctors and other medical personnel may not be as Lewy-savvy as you would like. This doesn't make them inept professionals—it simply means their information is spread broadly over many diseases compared to a care partner's narrower focus on a single one. Learn all you can—and keep on learning. Care partners often find themselves teaching the professionals, or working as a team with them.

Our doctor is very supportive and I am so glad we found her. However, sometimes I feel like we should be charging her instead of paying her. My husband was one of her first known MCI-LB patients and she admits she is learning along with us. I do a lot of research and share it all with her. It has helped us get better care though. I'm actually very glad she's so open to new information. — Joyce

Knowledge may not come easily. Newcomers to the idea of LBD often report that books and articles about the disorder are painful to read. The content can be frightening or even anger-making. Care partners may not want to be reminded that dementia is an issue that may have to be dealt with, perhaps in the near future. Few are ready to face challenges the future may bring. Take it slowly. Read a little. Take a break and then read some more. Talk about what you read. That is one of the best ways of retaining the information and making it less frightening.

Symptoms often confused by families and even the medical community:

Active Dreams: Dramas acted out while asleep. Seldom remembered after awaking, but may be thought real if they are remembered.

Hallucinations: Perceptual errors where the person sees, hears or otherwise senses something that isn't truly real.

Delusions: Thinking errors where the person believes something that isn't really true. Often expressed as dramas acted out while awake and usually remembered for hours, days or weeks.

Illusions: Perceptual errors where something is really there, but the person sees it incorrectly.

Sundowners: Increased confusion and agitation in the evenings. Can include hallucinations, illusions or delusions.

Chapter 1

The Lewy Body Family

To understand how LBD is connected to other disorders, it helps to know how it starts out in the brain. LBD affects the whole body. However, that's not why it is called Lewy "body" dementia. It was named after Dr. Frederic Lewy who first discovered microscopic round bodies, or deposits, in the brain. Later researchers found that the deposits were made of misfolded alpha-synuclein proteins that clump together and become toxic.[4]

Although researchers are unsure about what causes improper folds, they currently believe that in most cases, genetic and environmental factors interact to cause Lewy body disorders.[5] Genetics alone accounts for only a small amount of the cases. Likewise, simple exposure to environmental toxins is seldom enough. When the genetics and exposure to toxins such as herbicides and pesticides combine, the chances of developing a Lewy body disorder greatly increase.[6]

Some toxins are more dangerous than others. Perhaps the most well-known is Agent Orange, a chemical used in the Vietnam war. The US government has decreed that a military person developing certain neurological problems, including Parkinson's and Lewy body dementia, after exposure to Agent Orange is eligible for medical benefits.[7] Not all persons exposed to Agent Orange developed neurological problems—support for the theory that one must also carry the "susceptibility" genes.

> *Misfolded proteins:* A protein structure that does not fold properly becomes nonfunctional, or like Lewy bodies, toxic.
>
> *Lewy bodies:* Misfolded alpha-synuclein proteins that clump together into microscopic round deposits.
>
> *Neurotransmitters:* Chemicals that neurons (brain cells) use to communicate with other neurons.

Unlike the damaged Alzheimer's-related proteins, which are found mainly in the cerebral cortex, Lewy bodies reside in many areas of the brain. However, Lewy bodies are more selective, attacking neurons that contain certain neurotransmitters. The targeted chemicals vary, depending on the area of the brain. The attacked neurons weaken, become unable to function properly and eventually die.[8]

Although it is presently impossible to identify Lewy bodies except by autopsy, more advanced brain scans may eventually be able to show them. Researchers also have found Lewy bodies in other areas of the body, including the gastro-intestinal tract where detection is easier (e.g., with a sample of intestine taken during a routine colonoscopy).[9]

Besides dementia, these microscopic bodies are present with motor problems, autonomic nervous system dysfunctions, perceptual problems, mood disturbances and more. The symptoms depend on where the damaged proteins are located in the brain.

Lewy Body Disorders

In the *Guide*, we recognized three disorders caused by Lewy bodies, i.e., Lewy body disorders:

Parkinson's Disease (PD). In the mid-brain, Lewy bodies affect brain cells that make dopamine, which is needed for fine motor control. This results in the motor symptoms of Parkinson's disease. Although PD starts out as a movement disorder, other symptoms appear as the disease progresses. One of the most distressing is dementia.

Lewy Body Dementia (LBD). While this term was once synonymous with dementia with Lewy bodies (DLB), it is now an umbrella term that defines both types of dementia caused by Lewy bodies: DLB and Parkinson's disease with dementia (PDD).

- *Dementia with Lewy Bodies.* Lewy bodies in the cerebral cortex target the chemical acetylcholine, causing cognitive losses to appear. When this occurs before Parkinson's, the resulting disorder is called dementia with Lewy bodies.
- *Parkinson's Disease with Dementia.* When someone with PD develops dementia, it usually means that the Lewy bodies have spread from the midbrain to the cortex. Both dopamine and acetylcholine are targeted, which causes both motor and dementia symptoms. Parkinson's Disease with Dementia is the second type of LBD.

Earl has had Parkinson's for five years and we never heard that it had anything to do with Lewy bodies—or Lewy body dementia. He has been having hallucinations for a year or so but Earl's doctor just told us that hallucinations are a symptom of PD and not to worry. We've been attending a PD support group for a couple of years and no one mentioned dementia or LBD there either, even when Earl talked about seeing things. — Julie

The truth is that while hallucinations do occur with Parkinson's, they are also early symptoms of dementia. Julie and Earl's experience was several years ago. Since then, that attitude is changing. There is a growing interest in the Parkinson's community about the non-motor effects of the disorder.

A ready-made group of people at risk for dementia, people with PD comprise most of the subjects in the growing pool of research about early and pre-LBD. It is important to remember that Lewy body dementia doesn't always start with Parkinson's. About half the time it skips the PD and goes right to dementia, which is then called dementia with Lewy bodies (DLB). Even so, the two types are so similar that almost everything researchers learn about PDD and its precursors can also be applied to DLB, and thus to LBD in general.

Two More Lewy Body Disorders

Since the *Guide* was published in 2010, research has added more to the list of disorders where Lewy bodies are always present in the brain.

Mild Cognitive Impairment-Lewy Body type (MCI-LB), also called non-amnestic MCI. The cognitive losses of this type of MCI include thinking, planning and other executive skills. A person may be able to remember names fairly well but their ability to do once easy tasks diminishes. If the disorder advances to dementia, it will usually be LBD rather than AD.[10]

REM Sleep Behavior Disorder (RBD), also called Active Dreams. Although RBD can occur alone, it is a very common precursor of PD and both types of Lewy body dementia. When researchers autopsied brains of people who died with RBD, they found Lewy bodies even when no other LB disorder was present.[11] Thus it is included here as a Lewy body disorder, usually the first one to appear. It is also very common with Multiple System Atrophy (MSA) discussed in the next chapter.

Chapter 2

Other Related Disorders

Some Lewy "cousins," are similar disorders and syndromes caused by damaged proteins other than Lewy bodies. Others are not so closely related but share many LBD symptoms and often appear with it. LBD appears alone only about 5% of the time. Autopsies usually show evidence of two or more dementias even when observable symptoms were specific to only one.

> *Syndrome:* A group of symptoms with a similar apparent cause and collective outcome. The third level of diagnostic clarity, after disease and disorder, the cause of a syndrome is usually uncertain.

It is understandable to be upset to learn that Lewy teams must deal with other disorders as well. All the names, each with its own alphabet of often similar sounding initials, might be confusing and even intimidating. Hang in there. As you become more knowledgeable, the disorders and acronyms will sort themselves out.

The Cousins

Although the following are not caused by Lewy bodies, their symptoms are so similar that they are often misdiagnosed as Lewy body disorders or even one of the look-alikes such as AD. This first one is believed to be caused by the same alpha-synuclein protein except that in this case, it is misfolded (damaged) differently. The others are believed to be caused by other damaged proteins in the brain.

Multiple System Atrophy (MSA),[12] caused by alpha-synuclein protein misfolded in a way differently than Lewy bodies, affects men and women equally, primarily in their 50's. Like Lewy body disorders, MSA attacks movement and the autonomic nervous system. Active Dreams occur in up to 90% of people with MSA. However, it rarely causes dementia or the perceptual symptoms such as delusions and hallucinations that lead to acting-out.[13]

Parkinson's Plus Syndromes (PPS). These are neurological conditions, believed to be caused by damaged proteins other than the alpha-synuclein proteins mentioned above. These syndromes are often misdiagnosed due to the following similarities to Lewy body disorders and to each other.[14]

- Symptoms such as slowness of movement, muscle rigidity, gait disturbances, irritability, apathy, personality changes, and cognitive difficulties.
- More common in men than women.
- Average onset in the mid-40s to mid 70's.
- A poor response to PD drugs. The diagnosing doctor will often start their patient on these drugs. If they do poorly, then they know they probably aren't dealing with PD.

Each syndrome has unique characteristics as well.

Corticobasal Degeneration (CBD).[15] This is believed to be caused by the damaged protein, tau. It affects nerve cells in the midbrain and cerebral cortex. Their degeneration results in the Parkinson's Plus symptoms plus poor balance and coordination, tremor, and speech difficulties. Motor symptoms may occur on only one side at first.

Progressive Supranuclear Palsy (PSP).[16] This also has brain shrinkage that results in the above Parkinson's Plus symptoms. While people with PSP generally have severe balance problems with frequent falls, they are usually able to stand straight (unlike PD, where a stooped posture is common). Speech and swallowing difficulties can be severe. Visual problems can also be severe, including light sensitivity, blurred vision and abnormal eye movements, although hallucinations (a hallmark for LBD) are uncommon. Resting tremor, common with PD, is rare with PSP.

The Look-alikes

Alzheimer's Disease (AD). It is difficult to talk about LBD without mentioning Alzheimer's. DLB is often diagnosed first as AD. In fact, until recently, it almost always was. Even PDD was diagnosed as Parkinson's with Alzheimer's until the late 1990's. Damaged proteins in the cerebral cortex first affect memory and, later, many other cognitive functions such as speech and complex thinking. Hallucinations, common early in LBD, seldom appear until in the later stages of AD.

Vascular dementia (VaD). A series of small strokes that deprive the brain of vital oxygen causes VaD. Symptoms, such as disorientation in familiar locations, walking with rapid, shuffling steps, incontinence, laughing or crying inappropriately, difficulty following instructions, and problems handling money may appear suddenly and worsen with additional strokes.

This type of dementia is not progressive. That is, each small stroke causes damage but it doesn't get worse unless another stroke occurs. However, the strokes can be very close together and the condition may appear to be progressive. Controlling risk factors such as high blood pressure, cigarette smoking, and high cholesterol, helps to prevent further episodes of this dementia.[17]

VaD often appears as a third dementia with AD and LBD in autopsies. It may not be recognized in life because the symptoms are so similar to other dementias. Even the stroke that caused it may go unnoticed by appearing as simply a few "bad" days, a fluctuation that is common to LBD.

Frontotemporal Dementia (FTD).[18] Although this disorder may be misdiagnosed as LBD, it is caused by different proteins. It is the most common dementia for people under 60 years of age—even more common than Alzheimer's. This disorder affects one's ability to empathize, making person with FTD appear unfeeling and selfish.

As with LBD, thinking errors and delusions are common. However, there are fewer physical or memory problems. This, along with its early onset, makes it difficult to identify and it is often diagnosed as depression or a personality defect the person is unwilling to change. Like LBD, it is more common in men.

Mixed Dementias

Alzheimer's is the most common dementia to accompany DLB, where the thinking problems start before motor problems. Although it can also accompany PDD, this is less frequent. When symptoms more specific to Alzheimer's occur, such as wandering or recent memory loss, it is probably because AD is actually present. VaD often accompanies either type of LBD. A sudden drop in functioning may herald its presence, especially if the functioning does not return to previous level. Frontotemporal dementia seldom accompanies LBD although early symptoms such as delusions can be very similar.[19]

Chapter 3

LBD Risk Factors

A person doesn't go directly from being perfectly healthy, or even from having Parkinson's to having dementia. It is a very gradual process that starts well before symptoms are noticeable. Our take on it is this: When enough Lewy bodies build up in an area, then symptoms related to that area appear. Actually, it isn't just the *number* of Lewy bodies that is important; it's the number of Lewy bodies *versus* the number of healthy brain cells. Symptoms appear when the reserve of healthy cells isn't enough to compensate for the damage that the Lewy bodies have caused.

LBD risk factors are indications that Lewy bodies may already be somewhere in the brain. They warn that eventually, enough of these damaged proteins may collect in the cerebral cortex to cause dementia symptoms. Most LBD risk factors are disorders such as PD or symptoms, such as hallucinations. While a Lewy team can seldom prevent risk factors initially, recognizing them as warning signs provides a head start for slowing down the disorder's progression towards dementia.

Risks factors are usually quantified by percentages and years. For example the risk for a person with PD to develop dementia by age 85 is 65-80%. These statistics are not set in stone; they are averages. Don't let them be frightening. Instead work to change the statistics for your team by using the preventative measures such as stress management, discussed later in this book. There's still a chance that dementia will appear but it will likely be later in life than it otherwise would have been.

Uncontrollable Risk Factors

Age is the most common risk factor for LBD. All studies show that with or without PD or any other factors, the risk for dementia increases with age. This does not mean that age causes Lewy bodies. However, Lewy bodies do increase with age. The older a person is, the more likely it is that the damaged proteins will become so numerous that symptoms appear.

Genetics or heredity accounts for about 10% of those diagnosed with Lewy body disorders.

Especially important is Gaucher's disease, an inherited metabolic disorder where lipids (fatty materials) accumulate in several organs of the body including the brain. The disease is caused by a mutation of the GBA gene. Although a person must have a copy of the mutated gene from each parent to get the disease, even a single mutation of the gene can increase the risk for both PD and LBD about five fold.[20]

Whatever the reason, if more than one family member has a Lewy body disorder, other family members may also be at risk. Such a family history increases the urgency to take care of yourself by living a healthy lifestyle, decreasing stress and avoiding certain types of drugs.

Symptoms or Disorders as Risk Factors

The following symptoms can show up early in the Lewy body journey:

- Parkinson's disease (PD)
- Mild cognitive impairment (MCI)
- REM sleep behavior disorder (RBD)—Active Dreams
- Mood disorders
- Autonomic nervous system disorders
- Increased sensitivity to certain drugs

It is not unusual to find many or even all of the above in the same person. No single symptom is linked 100% to LBD. The presence of a single symptom is only a warning which may never proceed to full-blown LBD. It depends on how big the reserve of healthy brain cells is, how well maintained that reserve is and how much it is assaulted by stress and other irritants. The chance of dementia also increases with the addition of more risk factors.

Chapter 4

Parkinson's Disease

Helen's sister Lucille had Parkinson's (PD). A retired schoolteacher, she had done her research and knew what might lie ahead for her.

When I became Lucille's caregiver, she warned me that dementia could be a PD symptom. Even though I had been a nurse for years, this was my introduction to Parkinson's disease with dementia (PDD)—I'd never heard of it before. Lucille told me, "So far I've been lucky. I'm a little slower than I used to be but otherwise, I don't think it's hit me--yet." She was right; she could still think clearly when she died at age 78. – Helen Whitworth

Helen and Lucille didn't know then how fortunate they were. Nancy and her husband, Del, were not so lucky.

Parkinson's Dark Secret

In 2006, Del was diagnosed with dementia. We were shocked. We'd been dealing with his Parkinson's for eight years—attending the support groups, listening to all those lectures—and yet, no one, not even Del's doctor, had mentioned dementia until that day. We thought we were coping, but this hit us hard. We weren't prepared. — Nancy

Graham Lennox called dementia "The dark secret of Parkinson's disease" in a 2006 presentation[21] he did at about the same time that Nancy and Del were struggling with his diagnosis. "Please spread the word," Nancy begs. "Don't leave other families in the dark as we were."

> *Parkinson's disease (PD):* A neurological disorder caused by Lewy bodies in the midbrain, where fine motor control is managed. Symptoms include tremors, muscle rigidity, posture imbalance, and other physical problems.
>
> *Parkinson's disease with dementia (PDD):* When Lewy bodies migrate to the thinking areas of the brain such as the cerebral cortex, dementia symptoms appear along with the Parkinson's symptoms.

The lifetime risk for dementia in the general public is less than 20%.[22] The risk for PwPD to develop dementia in their lifetime is 65-80%.[23] Even so, many remain unaware of this. Nancy and Del were blindsided by his doctor's announcement that Del had PDD. There were several reasons for their lack of information in 2006. As this book goes to print in 2015, these reasons still exist to some extent.

PDD is a "new" disorder. While it was known that dementia often accompanied PD, until the early 1990s, it was usually considered to be a separate disorder, likely Alzheimer's. In 1994, "Parkinson's disease with dementia" was included in the DSM-IV, the basic diagnostic manual for mental disorders, and added to the insurance codes. It usually takes two or three decades for awareness of a "new" disease to spread throughout the medical community.

Cross-sectional studies don't tell the true story. Although dementia has finally become recognized as a symptom of PD, Parkinson's websites often quote cross-sectional studies.

> *My doctor told me I had about a 30% chance of getting dementia. That's a lot less than the 65-80% you are quoting. How do you explain the difference? — Tyrone*

A cross-sectional study is a single "snapshot" of a specified group of people—in this case, people with PD at that time. These studies usually report a 20% to 30% rate of occurrence, numbers that make the possibility of impending dementia easy to ignore or deny. Cumulative studies, i.e., studies done of a group of people over time, show that 65-80% eventually develop dementia.

PD doctors are movement, not dementia, specialists. Until lately, neurologists who specialize in treating Parkinson's focused heavily on movement issues and were less likely to be trained to recognize early signs of PDD. When movement specialists saw signs of dementia, they tended to shrug them off as evidence that their patient had entered late-stage PD. In such cases, dementia often went untreated until it was so severe that it couldn't be ignored.

This is changing. A report from the 17th Annual International Congress on Parkinson's Disease and Movement Disorders (ICPMD) in June of 2013 states that there is a much greater incidence of mental deficits in Parkinson's than previously thought.[24] While *dementia* specialists have been making similar reports for several years, reports like this are new to the *movement disorder* community. These new reports have had an effect. Many forward thinking movement specialists are now very aware of the cognitive aspects involved.

The risk of dementia increases with age and duration of the disorder but it can occur as early as a year after the PD diagnosis. Additionally, recent studies have found that mild cognitive impairment, a major risk factor for eventual PDD, is often present in PD's early stages—even at diagnosis.

While anyone with PD is at risk for eventual dementia, the risk increases with:

Age of PD onset. Studies show that fewer people who get PD prior to age 50 will develop dementia than those who were diagnosed later in life.[25] This is good news for people like Michael J. Fox, diagnosed with PD at age 30. It isn't such good news for people like Nancy's husband, Del, diagnosed with PD in his 60's.

Duration of PD symptoms. At least 75% of those who survive for more than fifteen years past their PD diagnosis develop dementia.[26]

Chronological age. Dementia is most likely in people age 70 and older, increasing to 80% for those in their 80's.[27]

Other risk factors. The appearance of the risk factors named in this section, such as Active Dreams or MCI, increases the eventual likelihood of PDD. However, when they are already present *when PD is diagnosed,* dementia is likely to appear within 10 years or sooner.

Chapter 5

Mild Cognitive Impairment - LB

Mild cognitive impairment (MCI) precedes but does not always progress to dementia. In the past, this disorder has been associated with Alzheimer's, and a diagnosis had to include memory loss. In the last decade, researchers have found that it can also start with a loss of executive abilities such as complex thinking, planning and doing sequential tasks.[28]

Mild cognitive impairment (MCI): Cognitive losses not severe enough to significantly interfere with functional tasks or activities of daily living. Must include at least some loss of executive function or memory.

Mild cognitive impairment—amnestic type (MCI-AD): MCI associated with Alzheimer's and characterized by recent or short term memory loss.

Mild cognitive impairment—non-amnestic type (MCI-LB): MCI caused by Lewy bodies and characterized by losses of executive functions more than memory. In this book "MCI" means "MCI-LB" unless otherwise stated.

This disorder can occur alone or with other symptoms that warn of eventual LBD, including DLB, the type that starts without motor symptoms. However, most of the research involving MCI-LB is with people who already have PD.

Parkinson's never interfered with my work. I'm an accountant. That's a job that uses brain rather than brawn and my brain was fine. Well, it was until a while back. First thing I noticed was that I couldn't seem to keep my paperwork straight and filing was, well, awful—I just couldn't do it. When I realized that even simple math had become confusing, that's when I went to the doctor. He told me I had some mild cognitive impairment. I didn't agree. I didn't have any trouble remembering names and such. I was sure he was wrong. But then, he said it wasn't that kind of MCI. It was the kind that comes with Parkinson's. — Arlene

Most people are like Arlene. They consider Parkinson's a motor disorder rather than a cognitive disorder. However, new research is showing that mild cognitive impairment can accompany it right from the beginning:[29]

- MCI occurs in up to 40% of newly diagnosed PD patients and over 65% of all PwPD meet the criteria for MCI.
- The chance of eventual dementia increases when MCI is present at or near a PD diagnosis.
- The chance of eventual dementia increases even more when, in addition to MCI, other risk factors are also present at or near a PD diagnosis.

A person with MCI-LB may have only one of the following symptoms (single domain) or several (multiple domain):

Executive function. These include difficulties with problem-solving, initiating and planning, multitasking, sequencing, impulse control, following through and monitoring performance.

Memory. Memory retrieval may become difficult. This may include tasks learned long ago—playing the piano, using electrical equipment, driving or even brushing one's teeth. Learning new information is still possible with adequate repetition. (This is different from MCI-AD where the memory loss pertains more to words, people and places rather than tasks.)

Mental processing. Processing and responding to information slows down. This has a domino effect that can impair other cognitive abilities, including problem-solving and memory retrieval.

> *MCI steals into my brain and slows it down, way down, and then it stirs things around and makes it difficult for me to think clearly. Everything is still possible. It's just so much harder and I get confused so much easier. — Lester*

Language fluency. Finding the proper word to use becomes difficult (it's on the tip of my tongue syndrome).

> *MCI can also steal words, so that I can't find the right one although I can still describe it and can usually find an alternate word that will work. – Lester*

Attention. Maintaining focus on a task becomes difficult and getting off-track more likely.

Multi-tasking. Trying to do more than one thing at a time or deal with more than one choice or idea may become frustrating and stressful.

Sequencing: Doing a series of tasks becomes difficult. Most tasks are actually a series of smaller tasks. Tooth brushing consists of finding the right toothbrush, opening the toothpaste, putting it on the brush, etc., etc.

Visual-spatial abilities. Perceiving, processing and acting on visual information becomes difficult. This impairs driving, reaching or walking.

MCI-LB, unlike the amnestic, pre-AD MCI, may accelerate abruptly. Such a sudden change is often triggered by a stressful event such as illness, injury or surgery, usually combined with a reaction to drugs that were used during the event. Then new, harder to manage LBD symptoms such as increased confusion, hallucinations or delusions may appear.

Chapter 6

REM Sleep Behavior Disorder (Active Dreams)

During normal dreams, a chemical toggle preserves rest by preventing most non-essential physical movement. Because this stage of sleep is associated with rhythmic eye movements, it is called Rapid Eye Movement (REM) sleep. When that switch is damaged, the resulting disturbance is called REM sleep behavior disorder (RBD). Care partners often use the term "Active Dreams" to describe these physically acted out dreams that can include talking, thrashing limbs about and even violent striking out at a bed partner.[30]

Sleep disorders are common with all dementias. However, RBD occurs with Lewy body dementia so often that it is included in the diagnostic criteria. Because Lewy bodies are found in brain autopsies of people with RBD who had neither PD nor LBD, it can be considered another Lewy body disorder.

Active Dreams may appear decades prior to any signs of dementia, or even Parkinson's disease. Just as a disorder can advance from Parkinson's disease into PDD, a disorder can go from RBD to Parkinson's and on to dementia. A person can also go directly from having Active Dreams to displaying symptoms of dementia with Lewy bodies. The presence of RBD at a Parkinson's diagnosis increases the chances of eventual dementia. When cognitive impairment is also present at that time, dementia is likely to appear within four years.[31]

I'm 57 and I've been experiencing Active Dreams since my late thirties. When the doctor diagnosed me recently with PD,

36

she also did some tests for MCI and found that my thinking ability was below normal. I'm not sure I believe her--I don't feel any different mentally. Well, a little slower maybe, but I can still do my checkbook and drive. – Roger

I'm 64 and I also received a Parkinson's diagnosis at 57. I know what you mean about Active Dreams too—I've had them for years—long before I had PD. I know that these dreams are part of the criteria for LBD and so I asked my neurologist to do some testing last month. I'm pleased to report that my scores are still in the normal range for my age. – Mary

Roger and Mary both had Active Dreams before they developed PD. However, Roger also has some MCI, which makes him a candidate for early dementia, even though it isn't problematic yet. Remember, a person who has RBD when diagnosed with Parkinson's is at risk for dementia in the *near* future *only* if there is MCI as well. While Mary's PD may go on into PDD eventually, it isn't as likely to do so for many years.

Of course, a person may never have Parkinson's. Annie, Jim's first wife, went from Active Dreams to DLB.

Five years before Annie started acting confused, she had Active Dreams. She talked and thrashed about. Once she tried to hit me. I teased her about that the next morning but she didn't remember it at all. — Jim Whitworth

People seldom remember their Active Dreams. However, when they do remember, the dreams feel very real.

Annie would dream that the doorbell was ringing and wake up demanding that I answer the door. She couldn't settle down and go back to sleep until I did. Of course, there was never anyone there. — Jim Whitworth

Clonazepam, a member of the benzodiazepine family, is the drug of choice for treating RBD. However, if MCI is present, this may not be safe as it can dull thinking. Drug sensitivities increase as LBD becomes more likely. The supplement, Melatonin, has been used with some success and fewer problems. Although neither of these drugs cures RBD, they may decrease the symptoms and improve sleep—a valuable result in itself.

Chapter 7

Mood Disorders

Mood disorders can occur alone or with many other neurological diseases such as AD and thus are not considered LBD risk factors when alone. When mood disorders are accompanied by at least one other risk factor, such as MCI-LB, they may be Lewy body related. As such, they predict an increased chance of dementia in the future.

Although depression and apathy are often partners, they are actually separate symptoms. Both frequently occur with Parkinson's disease, Mild cognitive impairment and Lewy body dementia. One or both can appear before tremors or other PD symptoms, and can be among the first symptoms of MCI or LBD.

Depression

Depression changes one's mood, thinking, physical well-being and behavior. It generates feelings of sadness, misery, unhappiness, anger, loss and frustration. Besides decreasing quality of life, it adds stress, and decreases one's ability to deal with illness.[32]

Performing tasks, making decisions or interacting with others all become more difficult when depression is present. Since these are also skills affected by dementia, it is sometimes difficult to tell if the symptoms are related to depression, dementia, or both. Of course, depression in a person with dementia can make already impaired skills even worse.

Depression is an understandable response to such life-changing news for the PwLB and care partner alike. This situational type is usually short term. With time, and treatment if needed, it can improve and eventually disappear.

When the depression doesn't leave, or appears to get worse, it may be organic, a neurological symptom of the disorder. Ongoing situational depression is also common with care partners and can last a long time. While not organic, it is a response to the continual bombardment of new responsibilities, new losses and feelings of inadequacies. Situational and organic depression can both be treated with antidepressants that tend to be safe with LBD.

Depression is common with many other diseases and neurological disorders, including Alzheimer's. However, it is so much more common with LBD that, in combination with other risk factors, it can be used to help with a diagnosis. When depression is present with MCI, a person is 50% more likely to advance to dementia than if depression were not present.[33]

Depression seriously affects one's quality of life. Anytime this symptom is present, the Lewy team should seek treatment. It can often be alleviated by the less Lewy-sensitive drugs, psychological treatment or both.

Apathy

Apathy is the lack of motivation, without associated feelings of depression. It damages one's self-starter—that extra push needed to overcome the inertia of inactivity. As it increases, it decreases the ability to keep going as well. With apathy, nothing is easy. Everything takes effort, often more effort than a person can muster up. Apathy is common with PD, and often appears with depression. When a PwPD has both MCI and apathy, dementia is apt to follow within three years.[34] However, there are many things you can do that will improve quality of life and may even extend the time before dementia appears.

The doctor can test to see if the PwPD has MCI or not. Many Lewy teams would just as soon not know for sure what their future holds. That's understandable. If you choose against the test, then assume the worst and hope for the best. Prepare for eventual dementia but do everything you can to slow the process.

If the care partner doesn't understand that apathy is a neurological symptom not under the person's control, this symptom may seem like giving up.

Henry has always been a take-action guy. Even when he was diagnosed with PD, he didn't let that stop him. He was a writer and he continued to write. When his tremor made typing difficult, he learned how to use a speech program. He was always physically active and he continued to be, even after PD put him in a wheelchair. Then I realized that he'd changed. He used to turn out pages of writing every day. Now he was turning out a few pages a week—if that. I couldn't remember the last time he'd had me take him to the gym. I thought he'd given up and I got mad. What gave him the right to give up when I was so affected too—I'd given up my job to care for him, after all. When I talked to the doctor about what I considered his reneging on life, he explained that Henry's apathy was a symptom of his disorder and not

*something that he could control. I felt so guilty then. —
Mabel*

Mabel's angry reaction is not unusual. Most caregivers would prefer to believe that what is happening to our loved one is controllable. Her guilt is understandable too. It's the first reaction most of us experience after accusing someone unfairly. Guilt can be as damaging as the apathy but fortunately, Mabel isn't stuck with it. Unlike Henry's apathy, which is organic or "hard-wired" and not under his control, Mabel's guilt is her response to a situation. She chose that response and she can choose to let it go.

Chapter 8

Autonomic Nervous System Dysfunctions

Lewy bodies may attack the autonomic nervous system (ANS) anytime from years before any PD is apparent to well after dementia has set in. As with most LBD risk factors, no ANS symptom alone can predict dementia. However, when the symptom appears in concert with symptoms in other areas of the body, such as Active Dreams or mood disorders, they help to nail down a LBD diagnosis.

Dysphagia

Dysphagia, or difficulty swallowing, may begin well before any cognitive symptoms do. When a person breaths, air travels down the throat and into the windpipe. When a person eats or drinks, food travels the same path down the throat but is shunted into the esophagus and on down into the stomach.

> *I've noticed that Arthur is having more trouble eating lately. He chokes more. He used to love sandwiches but now he says he doesn't like them anymore. I think it is because that's what usually makes him choke. Drinking isn't as easy as it used to be for him either. -- Belinda*

Arthur is showing classic signs of dysphagia.[35] Because his food is too dry to swallow easily, some goes "down the wrong pipe," into the windpipe instead of the esophagus, where they become "foreign substances" that can be harmful if allowed to travel further. His choking and coughing is his body's gag reflex, a normal response to this danger. So far, it has worked. He has been able to dislodge the foreign substances from his windpipe. Even so, choking and gagging can spoil the enjoyment of a meal and can be painful if it is intense. As Arthur's disorder progresses, aspiration will be become more of a danger. With aspiration, inhaled particles of food or drink travel to the lungs where they can cause pneumonia and even death.

> *Dysphagia.* Difficulty swallowing.
>
> *Throat (Pharynx):* Common channel for air and food.
>
> *Esophagus:* Connects the throat with the stomach.
>
> *Windpipe (Trachea):* Connects the throat with the lungs.
>
> *Aspiration:* Accidental inhaling of food particles or fluids into the windpipe and down into the lungs.
>
> *Gag reflex:* Normal response of choking and coughing due to threatened aspiration.
>
> *Aspiration pneumonia:* Infection and swelling of the lungs due the inhalation of a foreign substance.

Two ANS dysfunctions combine to cause Arthur's dysphagia and increase the possibility of aspiration. First, ANS controlled salivary glands may not secrete adequate saliva, which can make dry food such as the bread in his sandwiches too dry to swallow easily. Secondly, some of his throat muscles are controlled by the ANS. As these weaken and become less functional, swallowing is harder and coughing is weaker.

Speech therapists can help Arthur learn methods for safer swallowing and exercises and for strengthening his throat muscles.

Orthostatic Hypotension

Orthostatic hypotension (OH) often appears early enough to be included in the MCI-LB picture. Lewy bodies attacks and weakens the autonomic nervous system, which controls blood flow. Thus, when a person susceptible to OH gets right up from a lying or sitting position, the heart may be unable to pump adequate oxygen-carrying blood to the brain. This temporary loss of oxygen results in dizziness, fainting, or even falling.

At other times, the same person's blood pressure may be normal or it might even be high. Like depression, orthostatic hypotension alone does not indicate the presence of MCI although it can indicate the possibility of a LB cousin, Multiple System Atrophy. When OH accompanies cognitive symptoms, it can help to confirm a diagnosis of the Lewy body type of MCI vs. the type that occurs prior to Alzheimer's.

> *Several years ago, Aaron started falling down and we couldn't figure out why. "I just felt dizzy, and then I was on the floor," he told me. We thought it might be something he ate, or his eyes, or not enough sleep. We certainly never suspected low blood pressure--Aaron has had high blood pressure for years. We went to the doctor who had Aaron lie down on the exam table for a half hour and then sit up and have his blood pressure taken. We were amazed—it was really low! But then, when the doctor took it again in 10 minutes, it was back to normal. The doctor told us Aaron had low blood pressure on rising. — Jeanette*

Aaron's problem is a common Lewy symptom. Because the OH appeared prior to any mental issues, Aaron was able to deal with it himself. He simply sat down and waited ten minutes so that his blood pressure could stabilize enough to pump adequate oxygenated blood up into his brain. Then he could get up and move around without a problem. There are medications that are seldom likely to cause Lewy-sensitivity that can help too. Read more about OH and its medications in the *Guide*, starting on page 153.

> *The doctor didn't prescribe OH drugs for Aaron. He said they might interfere with Aaron's high blood pressure medications. Looking back, I think those episodes of low blood pressure were Aaron's first LBD symptoms. They started a couple of years before we became concerned about his forgetfulness and so we didn't connect it to the disorder until later. I have to watch Aaron like a hawk now—he forgets that he has to wait before he walks across the room! — Jeanette*

A person with LBD can have many other health issues, such as Aaron's chronic high blood pressure. These may make what would normally be a very safe medication unwise for that particular person.

As a LB disorder progresses into dementia, OH becomes more difficult to handle. The PwLBD may not remember that waiting between sitting up and walking is necessary. Therefore, the care partner must monitor the situation carefully.

Chronic Constipation

The ANS controls the functioning of the gastrointestinal (GI) tract. When it doesn't function well, digestion gets sluggish and chronic constipation can occur. Everyone occasionally has infrequent or hard-to-pass bowel movements. This is seldom anything to worry about. Changing one's eating habits to foods with more fiber and drinking plenty of fluids usually solves the problem. When the blockage is ongoing and simple remedies don't work, there may be a bigger problem. Sometimes medication can cause constipation. When changing the medication doesn't help, then it may be Lewy body related.

Chronic constipation is a common Lewy symptom, a neurologic problem not easily solved with changed eating habits or laxatives. In fact, overuse of laxatives can bring about early incontinence. A person with any Lewy body disorder who suffers chronic constipation should be tested for neurologic bowel syndrome. If it is present, he should be offered a bowel management program that fits his specific needs.[36]

This problem can show up very early in a person's life. It is not a common symptom of the amnestic, pre-Alzheimer's type of MCI but is often listed as a symptom of MCI-LB and Parkinson's.

> *Annie, my first wife, had chronic constipation for years. She'd learned to deal with it but when a physician told her that the problem could be fixed with surgery, she was thrilled. A few months after her surgery, she was diagnosed with mild dementia. — Jim Whitworth*

Annie did not have PD, but she did have a history of Active Dreams. That, combined with her long term chronic constipation, put her at serious risk for eventual LBD, along with its sensitivities to drugs, including those used in surgery. This was the 1990's, when few neurologists and even fewer physicians knew about the disorder. See Chapter 9 for more about drug sensitivities.

Urinary Tract Infections

Although urinary tract infections (UTIs) are rare in MCI, they do occur and can be serious. It pays to be alert for any sign of their presence. UTIs occur when bacteria enters the urinary tract. Poor hygiene is often a culprit, but even with the best of care, these infections become very common as dementia increases. This is especially true with LBD because of its ANS involvement.[37]

The ANS controls the bladder and all of the sphincters of the body. When the sphincters don't function properly, fluid may stagnate in the bladder and provide a home for bacteria. Then the backed up fluid offers a route for the bacteria to travel up the urinary tract to the kidneys. This can be life threatening.

> *George is a bit slower and he can't do some of the stuff he used to be able to do, like the bill paying. Most of the time he is so normal that I forget he has LBD but last month we had a scare. George started having a lot more hallucinations and Active Dreams. Then a couple of days later, he complained of pain in his gut and said that it hurt when he peed. I took George to the doctor and sure enough, it was a urinary infection. The doctor prescribed some medication for it and voila! George's hallucinations stopped! We were so relieved. You can bet that the next time George starts seeing things that I don't, I'll get him to the doctor right away. I won't wait for the physical symptoms. — Janice*

Janice and George's experience with his UTI is typical. Normal symptoms are pain, discomfort or blood when passing urine and lower abdominal pain. However, Lewy symptoms often increase first, as they did for George. Infections stress the body and exploit resources normally used to keep these symptoms in check. Care partners often suspect the presence of an infection before their loved ones do because they see the behavior more clearly. Janice now knows what to expect and she will think "UTI" the next time George begins acting erratically. There probably will be a next time; these infections become a fact of life for a Lewy team, even with the best of care.

Adequate fluids are extremely important for helping to prevent UTIs and cranberry juice seems to help. However, nothing provides 100% prevention. Once the infection is present, preventative methods are not adequate. Medication is needed.

Luckily, UTIs can be treated with medications that are seldom Lewy-sensitive. Once the infection is treated, the increased symptoms will usually recede.

Summary:

Dysphagia: Difficulty swallowing can be a fairly early symptoms. Can be treated with speech therapy.

Orthostatic Hypotension (OH): Low blood pressure on rising. Can start even before MCI. Can be treated with lifestyle changes (waiting before walking) and medications with low probability of Lewy-sensitivity.

Chronic constipation: Can appear very early in life. Better treated with lifestyle changes and gentle stool softeners than with surgery or more severe laxatives.

Urinary Tract Infections (UTIs): Even more common with Lewy body disorders than with other neurological diseases. Good personal hygiene, adequate hydration and home remedies such as cranberry juice can help to *prevent* UTIs.

Warning: Once a UTI is present, home remedies aren't strong enough to *cure* it. Consult the doctor at the first sign of a urinary tract infection. Do not wait. The sooner treatment starts, the better.

Chapter 9

The Problem with Drugs

There is no drug that actually treats a Lewy body disorder. Therefore, a person usually takes a variety of drugs to treat various symptoms. Some drugs, such as Exelon or Aricept, treat the dementia. These have been shown to be helpful while being generally safe with LBD.

Drug sensitivity: The reaction to a normal dose as though it were an overdose—sometimes a huge overdose, or with an adverse reaction. This response to certain drugs is a hallmark symptom of Lewy body dementia. Sensitivities can range from mild to severe, depending on the drug and the individual person's reaction to it.

Lewy-sensitive drug: One that may cause drug sensitivity or have an adverse reaction with LBD. These drugs will vary with each patient although some drugs are more likely to be Lewy sensitive than others.

Other drugs may be prescribed to treat symptoms such as low blood pressure upon rising, incontinence, constipation, or difficulty swallowing. Some of these drugs are safer with LB disorders than others. A Lewy-savvy physician will usually be aware of which are which and how to use them. However, not all medical personnel are Lewy-knowledgeable. Therefore, it is important to be prepared with adequate information about how these drugs interact with your loved one's disorder.

This chapter is very long. It wasn't going to be at first. After all, the *Guide* covers this subject well. However, all of the LBD caregivers who read the first draft insisted that it be expanded. They said that drug sensitivity is the most troublesome and feared part of this disorder. They wanted everyone dealing with LB disorders to know about these dangers right from the first. Those caregivers were right. However, the information in the *Guide* is still important. It provides an overview of Lewy-sensitive drugs used for conditions common to PwLB and suggests some safer choices.

Even with Parkinson's there can be some drug sensitivity. However, as Lewy bodies increase, so does the likelihood of drug sensitivity. The advent of even mild dementia makes this very serious symptom even more likely.[38] This sensitivity and avoiding its sometimes disastrous results becomes a major focus for most Lewy teams. However, learning about which drugs are safe and which aren't can seem daunting. It doesn't have to be. It is important to do your research and learn as much as you can about the drugs prescribed for the your loved one but the bottom line is fairly simple:

Be wary of any drug suggested to sedate or to treat anxiety or behavior-related problems. When used, be alert for signs of sensitivity (overdose or adverse reaction).

Ask the doctor or pharmacist about possible side effects of a drug given for any other problem such as bladder control and monitor closely. Pharmacists have more time to explain and often more expertise concerning drugs—that's their specialty.

Report any odd reactions to the doctor, especially those that cause or increase LBD symptoms, muscle problems or heavy sedation.

Ask about possible alternative therapy solutions to the problem. Many behavior issues respond well to non-drug anxiety and stress management.

The elderly in general are at risk for drug sensitivity.[39] Just as children require lower doses of medication than adults, so do the elderly. With age, the ability to metabolize drugs decreases and toxic levels build up quickly. Add LBD and the risk of sensitivity increases.

Any drug unsafe for use with LBD is also potentially dangerous for those *at risk for LBD*. Once a person has another Lewy body disorder like Parkinson's or Active Dreams, the same concerns apply. While the danger is less, an over-reaction to a drug may be the first LBD symptom noticed.

Lewy-sensitive drugs are those that most often cause or increase dementia symptoms in a person who is overly sensitive to them. These include:

- *Inhaled anesthetics*, used in surgery.
- *Anxiety and behavior* management drugs such as haloperidol (Haldol), clorazepate (Tranxene), diazepam (Valium) or alprazolam (Xanax).
- *Sleeping aids* such as zolpidem (Ambien), eszopiclone (Lunesta) or zaleplon (Sonata).

The following drugs are also troublesome, but less dangerous:

- *Cold and allergy medications* containing antihistamines, decongestants and benzodiazepines (ex: Robitussin DM, loratadine (Claritin) or diphenhydramine (Benadryl).
- *Opiates and other pain drugs* such as morphine or codeine.
- *Less safe ingredients* added to "safe" drugs such as acetaminophen (Tylenol) or aspirin. These combinations are often advertised as nighttime pain relievers.

Classifying Lewy-sensitive drugs can make them easier to identify. There are several ways to do this. One is to list the drugs by the properties or actions that make them dangerous:

Anticholinergic (anti-kol-en-er-gik) *action:* The drug blocks acetylcholine, a neurotransmitter needed for cognition. When Lewy bodies have already depleted this chemical, the drug may cause or increase *confusion and other dementia symptoms.*

Extrapyramidal (extra-pir-a-mid-al) *action:* The drug blocks dopamine, a neurotransmitter needed for mobility. When Lewy bodies have already depleted this chemical, the drug causes or increases *muscle stiffness, tremors, cramping, and constrictions.*

Sedative action: The drug slows down the central nervous system (CNS). When Lewy bodies have already comprised the autonomic part of the CNS, this causes *over-sedation or coma.*

The stronger the properties and the more of them present in a drug, the more likely that drug will be dangerous for a person with or at risk for LBD. For example, Atropine is a very strong anticholinergic and Haldol has all three properties. Both of these drugs are so likely to be dangerous in the presence of Lewy bodies that most Lewy-savvy doctors avoid their use with anyone at risk for LBD.

Another way to classify drugs is by type or drug family. Those of most concern are anticholinergics, antipsychotics, inhaled anesthetics and benzodiazepines.

Anticholinergics

Acetylcholine is a neurotransmitter that the brain needs to manage cognition. Anticholinergics are a huge class of acetylcholine-blocking drugs used to treat a variety of symptoms from anxiety to bladder control. These drugs should be used with caution, if at all, by the elderly and anyone at risk for dementia. The Resource Section in this book provides links to several published lists of these drugs. Review them and download the one you like the best to keep handy as a reference.

Antipsychotics

Antipsychotics (anti-sy-cot-iks) are a class of medications approved by the FDA to treat psychoses such as schizophrenia. Although they are not FDA-approved to treat dementia-related symptoms, doctors have been prescribing them to treat symptoms such as delusions, hallucinations, combativeness and disruptiveness for years. A person with Alzheimer's may appear to respond well but someone with LBD is more likely to respond poorly. All antipsychotics have a black label warning against use by the elderly or anyone with dementia because of a modest increased risk of death.

Traditional antipsychotics (TAs): Developed in the 1950's to treat severe psychosis, these drugs have strong sedative and extrapyramidal properties and less strong but still risky anticholinergic properties. Thus they can be quite dangerous when Lewy bodies are present. While most of these drugs are seldom used anymore, haloperidol (Haldol) is still used in hospital emergency rooms to calm down disruptive patients.

> *Maria had a fever and just wasn't acting right. It was the weekend and so I took her into the emergency room. The doctor said she was dehydrated—a problem she's had off and on before. When they tried to insert the IV, my wife began screaming that they were poisoning her. The nurse gave Maria a shot of Haldol. "We do this all the time with our dementia patients. It will calm her down so we can get some fluid in her," she told me. Well, Maria calmed down so much that they admitted her to the hospital. When she finally woke up ten hours later, her arms were drawn up to her chest and they stayed that way for weeks. It didn't seem to make her more confused, but I've heard it can do that too. — Renaldo*

The nurse was partially right. Until recently, Haldol has been considered comparatively safe for most people, including those with Alzheimer's—but it can be quite dangerous for someone at risk for Lewy body dementia. LBD caregivers have reported that even one regular dose caused:

- *extreme sedation*, as when their loved one remained unconscious for eight hours or more.
- *intense muscle constriction* that took over a week to relax.
- *confusion* that lasted for days, weeks or more.

Atypical antipsychotics: Also called second generation antipsychotics. These drugs don't cause the muscle problems that TAs can cause but do have strong sedative and anticholinergic properties. Many Lewy-savvy physicians still prescribe these drugs, especially Seroquel, as the best of the limited choices available for intervention with otherwise uncontrollable acting-out behaviors.

> ***Warning:*** Make sure the prescribing doctor is aware of the risks involved with most behavior and anxiety management drugs, including antipsychotics and benzodiazepines. Ask the physician if other less dangerous options are available. If not, ask if the prescribed dose is the smallest possible for the situation.

Benzodiazepines

Benzodiazepines (ben-zo-di-az-i-peens) are a family of sedative drugs with anticholinergic properties used to treat anxiety, insomnia and allergies. This combination makes them so potentially dangerous when Lewy bodies are present that they should be avoided or used with extreme caution. Drugs.com[40] provides an extensive list of these drugs along with their half-lives. The longer the half-life, the longer the drug will stay in the body. However, the presence of Lewy bodies tends to slow down the process and extend that time.

Benzodiazepine-based drugs may actually be unsafe for the elderly in general. A 2012 study of people ages 65 and over, found that those who had used benzodiazepines were 60% more likely to develop dementia in the next eight years than those who had never used these drugs.[41] While it is doubtful that benzodiazepines can *cause* LBD, this study shows that they may speed its appearance.

Anesthetics

Any drug strong enough to use for surgery will likely have the risk of being Lewy-sensitive. However, some are worse than others:

Inhaled anesthetics are gases such as isoflurane or enflurane used to induce a controlled coma and allow surgery.[42] These anesthetics often cause the elderly to be confused for several months after the procedure. Many LBD caregivers report that their loved ones remained confused after surgery and never returned to their pre-surgery level of cognition. Recent studies support this observation.[43]

Intravenous (IV) drugs such as midazolam (Versed), thiopental (Pentothal) or propofol (Diprivan) are not as Lewy-sensitive as inhaled drugs. Many LBD caregivers report successful surgeries using these drugs. That said, Versed is a strong benzodiazepine while Pentothal and Diprivan are a strong sedatives—both classes of Lewy-sensitive drugs.

Regional anesthetics "deaden" the area of the surgery. Used with spinal or epidural blocks, these anesthetics tend to be much safer than either of the above types of general anesthesia. Some major surgeries such as knee replacements can now be done with spinal or epidural blocks and low amounts of drugs such as propofol. A combination of regional anesthetics boosted by opiates or narcotics may also be used with these procedures. In either case, there appears to be less drug danger and less need for postoperative drugs.[44] Limitations include:

* This method is not for surgery in upper areas of the body, such as dental work.

- Because a person is awake during the procedure, cooperation is required. If the PwLB has a history of agitation during stress, this might not be an option.
- It requires an anesthesiologist skilled in the procedure. Most problems with this type of surgery result from it being done incorrectly.

Some of the danger from surgery can be avoided with a geriatric anesthesiologist who understands the sensitivity issues of the elderly.[45]

To help assure the best results with surgery:

- *Send a letter to the surgeon* well ahead of the surgery outlining your concerns. Include the LBDA wallet card and share any examples you have of your loved one's drug sensitivity. Ex: "Larry had hallucinations when he took Actifed for a cold."
- *Request a geriatric anesthesiologist.* If none are available, ask for an anesthesiologist who is either already Lewy-savvy or is willing to do some research about LBD and drugs prior to surgery. See Drug Alert Information and Forms in the Resources section for suggested readings.
- *Arrange to meet with the anesthesiologist prior to the surgery* to discuss your concerns about LBD and drug sensitivity. Share any examples you have of how the your loved one has responded to other drugs (as with the letter to the surgeon) to help the anesthesiologist judge drug sensitivity.

Other alternatives: In many cases, other options besides surgery are available—medication, physical therapy, or even learning to live with the problem. Where surgery might be the best solution for a healthy person, a non-surgical method might be the best for anyone with a Lewy body disorder. Be sure to ask about alternatives before agreeing to surgery.

Sometimes a person's first experience with drug sensitivity occurs after surgery:

> *Luke had very mild Parkinson's. He tripped and fell, breaking his leg. The doctor told us Luke would need surgery if he ever hoped to walk again but that with his PD, there was a possibility of dementia. So far Luke hadn't been particularly sensitive to any drugs and so we agreed to the surgery, mostly because he was in such pain. He started hallucinating in the recovery room, seeing bugs crawling on the walls. Then the delusions started and he became very frightened. He told me that he had to get out of the hospital. "There are some people in the room next door that are plotting to kill someone. They'll kill me if they know I heard them." I hoped that once he was home, and away from the hospital atmosphere, he'd improve. He did, some. But he still has times when he is very confused and he still has hallucinations now and then. We knew there was a chance of this, but we had to do it. We'd make the same decision again.*
> *— Cindy*

After major surgery, elderly people may have a period of "delirium," with symptoms similar to Luke's. With a healthy person, these symptoms can last for a few hours to as long as six months. When, as with Luke, Lewy bodies are already present, these symptoms may continue.

For Luke and Cindy, there was only one viable decision—have the surgery to stop the pain even if cognitive losses did show up afterward. For others it isn't that simple. In Chapter 8, Jim talked about Annie's chronic constipation.

The surgical "fix" the doctor suggested sounded like a no-brainer to us and so of course, she had the surgery. But then, not long afterward, I started receiving "burnt offerings" for dinner. No, she wasn't going off and forgetting it. She was right there, but she was turning the burner up instead of down. That was my first warning that things weren't right. A couple of months later, she was diagnosed with dementia. — Jim Whitworth

Annie's limited executive skills prevented her knowing which way to turn the knob for the effect she wanted. This made her unable to do a once familiar task, an early sign of LBD.

Prior to surgery today, Lewy-savvy doctors would check for risk factors like the Active Dreams Annie had had for several years. With her history, these doctors would probably recommend against the procedure. The drugs used during surgery probably didn't cause her dementia, but they may have lowered her reserves, allowing the symptoms to emerge sooner they otherwise would have.

If Annie had known what I know now about her risk for LBD, she would not have opted for her elective surgery. She had lived with this problem most of her life and she could have continued to do so. — Jim Whitworth

Sometimes the choice is between quality and length of life.

Bill's defibrillator battery was getting low and needed replacing, which required surgery. I asked the cardiologist if the device had been triggered. It hadn't, which made a decision against surgery easy. But then I found out his pacemaker battery was getting weak. It had been activated several times, making that decision harder. If the pacemaker quit, so would Bill's heart. I still decided against the surgery, opting for quality of life over quantity. The pacemaker functioned for two more years. When it stopped working, Bill died in his sleep. If I had it to do again, I'd make the same decision. — Marla

Consider all other options before surgery. If you decide that surgery is the best choice, try to use Lewy-knowledgeable surgeons and anesthesiologists even if it means traveling further from home. If this is not possible, ask the doctors involved to learn as much as they can bout LBD and drugs before they perform the surgery. See Drug Alert Information and Forms in the Resources section of this book for information to share with medical professionals.

Over-The-Counter (OTC) Drugs

Many cold and allergy drugs, which usually don't require a prescription, have benzodiazepines in their active ingredients. Less often, they have anticholinergics or sedatives. Any of these may trigger intense reactions, such as Active Dreams, hallucinations, delusions or general confusion. A Lewy team's first exposure to drug sensitivity may be with one of these OTC drugs.

I was diagnosed with RBD (Active Dreams) last fall. I'd sometimes wake up Jack but the dreams weren't serious and didn't seem to last long. For years, I've used a mild antihistamine for spring allergies with good results. When the allergies showed up last spring, I took my usual OTC allergy pill and went to bed. I had really scary dreams all night long. The next morning I found Jack on the sofa. He said I tried to attack him and so he escaped to the sofa. Of course, I didn't take any more of that drug and thankfully, the dreams reverted to their former benign state. — Shannon

As was the case for Shannon, reactions to these milder medications are seldom permanent. However, they can serve as a warning. People seldom know that they are sensitive to a drug until they take it and have a reaction--and then the damage may be done. Shannon and Jack have been forewarned. They can assume that she is also sensitive to other, more dangerous drugs and avoid them, thus eliminating the more serious problems they can cause.

With OTC drugs, the buyer takes on more responsibility. There's no doctor's prescription to tell you what to buy. You must choose from a shelf filled with similar drugs and hope it is the best one for the problem. Add Lewy's sensitivity issues, and the job gets even harder.

Learn to read labels. Avoid any drugs with active ingredients on the previously mentioned benzodiazepine or anticholinergic lists. The dangerous ingredients in OTC drugs will mostly likely be benzodiazepines. Check that list first.

Compare with known drugs. When you are unsure, find a medicine on the shelf that you know is unsafe. Compare the active ingredients of the compound in question with those of the known one. If the new medicine has some of the same ingredients, it is likely unsafe too.

Have a pharmacist you trust. Find a drug store with pharmacists familiar with LBD. Ask the pharmacist if your chosen medicines are compatible with Lewy body dementia.

Check with the doctor. It's a good idea to check with the doctor as well to make sure that a drug is not only safe with LBD but also with any other drug being taken. This is especially important when several doctors are involved. The movement specialist may not consider the drugs the cardiologist has prescribed. The cardiologist may forget about drugs the internist has prescribed. Always ask about compatibility.

Start small. A smaller than normal dose will very likely do the job and be less likely to cause problems.

Monitor carefully. Stop the drug immediately if unwanted symptoms appear and contact the prescribing physician.

Drug Sensitivity vs. Drug Allergy

Lewy bodies make people sensitive to drugs, not allergic to them. With allergies, that drug should be avoided altogether. With sensitivities, a smaller dose might be tolerated. Some drugs are too strong or too dangerous to take chances. Haldol and most sleep aids fit this category. Lewy-savvy physicians may consider experimenting with others, with these limitations:

- *The drug is considered mild.* Lorazepam (Ativan) and most OTC drugs fit this. Lewy-savvy physicians may prescribe a low dose of Ativan for anxiety or agitation.
- *Drug is short-acting,* i.e., rapidly absorbed, distributed and excreted. Atypical antipsychotics, most OTCs and many pain medications fit this.

- *Doses are small,* perhaps even a quarter of the normal amount. Tiny doses of pain medications like morphine may handle the pain with no unwanted side effects.
- *Careful monitoring.* Stop the drug as soon as unwanted symptoms appear.

Some people are so sensitive to drugs they would want to avoid all potentially Lewy-sensitive drugs.

Bud had some MCI but he was doing all right. Then he became very ill and got dehydrated. He started hallucinating and having delusions that made him pretty violent. The doctor gave him what she said was a mild anti-psychotic and it hit him awfully, constricting his muscles. He had been walking without even a cane before he got sick. Now he was almost bedridden. I couldn't care for him by myself and so I had to put him in a nursing home. He kept acting out and they kept medicating him. I finally convinced them to try taking him off all the drugs. It worked. He calmed down and his dreams stopped. But it took almost a month for Bud's muscles to relax. And even then, he was in a wheelchair. He was never able to walk again. — Jo

Bud's Lewy-related drug sensitivity was triggered by many drugs, even those that often help others with LBD. With any Lewy disorder, drugs should be started in *tiny* doses with increases until the effect wanted appears *or* there is a problem. Stop the drug at the first sign of a problem. It won't get better and will likely get worse.

Bud didn't recover right after the drugs were withdrawn. That's because Lewy bodies slow the normal process of flushing out the drugs. They were still in his system for a while, still causing reactions. The longer the drug-related symptoms last, the more likely it is that the patient will not be able to return to their previous level of functioning.

Because Lewy teams tend to be more aware of the dangers of these drugs than even many medical professionals, you need to be ready to act proactively, speak up to the medical community and insist on your rights.

In the Hospital

You may have a very knowledgeable neurologist, and an understanding primary physician. However, if you have a crisis and enter a hospital system, these supportive people won't be there. Instead you must deal with hospital personnel who may be less Lewy-savvy.

> *I took Annie to the ER when she had become dehydrated. She was hallucinating and agitated while they were infusing her with liquids. They gave her Haldol. When I voiced my concern, the nurse told me not to worry. "We do this all the time," she said. "It will calm her down." Annie calmed down so much that they couldn't wake her up and she had to be admitted to the hospital. — Jim Whitworth*

Annie's scenario is common when a PwLBD goes to the ER. Since LBD is worse during times of stress, hallucinations, delusions, and agitation become likely. Many ER units use antipsychotics like Haldol regularly for such behavior. Usually, they work well…just not with LBD. Since Annie's time, ER staff has become better trained but don't count on this. Be proactive—be prepared.

When Annie woke up in the hospital hours later, her muscles had tightened so that she couldn't move her arms. The hospitalist gave her something "to help her relax." Her arms did relax but she started hallucinating again. The doctor ordered ongoing doses of Haldol. Naturally, her muscles constricted again. Finally, he stopped the antipsychotic and changed to a different muscle relaxant. She stopped hallucinating and the rigidity gradually went away. — Jim Whitworth

When a person enters a hospital, they leave their personal doctors behind and deal with the hospital physician (hospitalist). Although the two physicians may eventually connect, responsibility for initial care is up to a hospitalist who may be less Lewy-savvy and therefore less likely to prescribe medications which may be Lewy-sensitive.

Annie died in 2003. She didn't have a Lewy-savvy physician or neurologist to provide support; that information was just beginning to appear. Today, you can have that support even in a hospital situation but you may have to make it happen. Put together an Emergency Room Kit.

Start by asking your loved one's doctor to write a note of explanation. With medical personnel, a note by a Lewy-savvy physician can be much more effective than any layman's words.

Obtain a free Medical Alert Wallet Card[46] from the LBDA. Carry it at all times and use it whenever you deal with medical personnel. Written in language medical personnel understand, it will likely be more acceptable than your layman's terms.

Write out any information specific to your loved one and keep it current. The stress of ER and hospital visits increases mistakes and forgetfulness for everyone, including the caregiver. Don't rely on memory alone.

List all current medications. Most medical teams want to know this right away. Using the form in the Emergency Room Kit provides other important information at the same time.

This form includes a warning about the danger of neuroleptic malignant syndrome (NMS) or catastrophic reaction.[47] This syndrome is quite rare but it is a possible reaction and its seriousness should get their attention! The drugs and drug families known to be Lewy-sensitive are already printed on the form. Add any others that have caused problems.

The form also includes a directive to consult a specified person (usually the care partner) before the introduction of any new medication. At such stressful times, the PwLB will seldom be in a condition to make decisions. However, *someone* who knows the dangers of mixing these drugs with LBD needs to be consulted. Using this form may prevent serious reactions and could even save lives. The *Guide*, pages 102-114, provides an overview of Lewy-sensitive drugs used for common conditions and suggests some safer choices.

Emergency Room Kit

Take these items on all medical errands. Have copies of documents placed in the PwLB's medical file. Find a downloadable copy of the ER Kit online at LBDtools.com/links.html.

LBDA Medical Alert Wallet Card.
(lbda.org/content/lbd-medical-alert-wallet-card)
Carry copies everywhere.

Hospital Form. (lbdtools.com/resources.html)

Health Care Directive. (uslwr.com/formslist.shtm)

Mental Health Directive.
(dbsalliance.org/advance_directives)

Treating Psychosis in LBD. (lbda.org/go/ER) An article to download and keep to give to ER staff.

Power of Attorney (naela.org) or other documents allowing the care partner to make decisions for the PwLBD.

Any letters of explanation from Lewy-savvy physicians.

Your daily journal, with appropriate entries bookmarked.

Distractions, such as finger food or MP3 player and ear buds.

Alternatives to Behavior Management Drugs

Lewy teams experience a catch-22 situation. LBD symptoms cause many difficult behaviors and yet most behavior management drugs are not safe with this disorder. However, there are alternatives.

Difficult behavior:

- Is often a stress-related form of communication that will decrease when the underlying message is identified and dealt with.
- Is easier to prevent than manage.
- Often responds well to alternative therapies such as massage or aromatherapy.

Use this information to reduce the need for drugs. For more information about stress and communication, see Sections Three and Four.

Summary

Drug sensitivity occurs when a person reacts to a normal dose of a drug as though it were an overdose or with an adverse reaction.

Avoid drugs that act to limit acetylcholine, such as antipsychotics, anti-anxiety drugs and OTC medicines.

Side effects that indicate drug sensitivity include muscle rigidity, extreme sedation, increased confusion and other Lewy body symptoms with resulting acting-out.

The effects of some drugs may be long lasting. Symptoms will last until the drug leaves the body. This may take weeks or even months. The longer it takes, the more likely some of the symptoms will remain.

Start any medication at a very low level and increase it slowly until you get the desired effect or negative effects appear.

Carry a LBDA Medical Alert card at all times. Also include a notice that describes personal sensitivities and designates a certain person as spokesperson.

Try non-drug intervention before resorting to behavior management drugs. This usually means identifying the stress-related message the behavior is meant to convey and responding to the need, often with some kind of alternative therapy.

Reminder: The authors of this book are not physicians. They are caregivers and report what they and other caregivers have learned by experience, and from physicians and literature. Always consult a physician about individual issues.

Chapter 10

Early Signs of LBD

The earliest Lewy body dementia symptom for each person will vary with the person, just as all symptoms do. Many are also signs of other Lewy body disorders, symptoms like the "it's on the tip of my tongue" syndrome of MCI-LB, the thrashing about of Active Dreams, or the hallucinations of Parkinson's. Others are symptoms that also accompany Parkinson's, such as chronic constipation or the dizziness that comes from low blood pressure on rising but are also symptoms of LBD.

One sub-type of dementia with Lewy bodies (DLB) starts with behavioral symptoms rather than cognitive losses—or along with them. These symptoms cause an apparently healthy person to behave in a way that seems "abnormal" and often, considered unacceptable.

At a Caregiver Support Group:

Laura: Dick's been forgetful for a while—but then that happens to all of us as we age. But now, he's getting mad at the oddest things. It just wasn't like the man I'd known for years. I talked him into going to the doctor who referred us to a specialist. We were both surprised when she diagnosed Dick with non-amnestic mild cognitive impairment. She explained to us that it wasn't the Alzheimer's type. She said it was the kind of MCI that's related to Parkinson's and can go on to become Lewy body dementia. My Aunt Mary has Parkinson's and she can hardly walk. Dick walks just fine.

Janet: Your doctor is right. But there are a couple kinds of LBD. One shows up after Parkinson's has set in and the other shows up before. Maybe Dick has the before kind.

Laura: My doctor also said that Dick's acting funny was probably a symptom of the LBD.

Janet: What do you mean by acting funny?

Laura: Well, he's driven away most of our friends with his irrational fits of anger. Oh, and he sees things no one else sees. It's really frustrating.

Janet: Yes, that sounds like LBD, all right. My mother's doctor told us that acting-out is a lot more common with LBD than with Alzheimer's.

Behavioral symptoms may appear before cognitive symptoms. Hallucinations and delusions are signs of impaired thinking ability and warn that more than MCI is occurring; dementia is on its way.[48] Remember that MCI means "cognitive losses not severe enough to significantly interfere with functional ability or activities of daily living." These symptoms, especially delusions, can cause major interferences with daily living.

Once behavior symptoms are present, tests will often find other, more conventional cognitive impairment. As these cognitive symptoms grow, you may also see fluctuations. Hallucinations may grow worse and cause concern, then seem to improve, or even disappear, only to return—sometimes the next day or the next month. This signifies a Lewy body disorder, rather than another type of dementia like Alzheimer's. These symptoms may last for a period of months or years and then quit, or may continue throughout the rest of the journey.

After a year in which I recorded eight delusions, five wanderings, twelve hallucinations, and numerous falls, those incidents stopped. One early morning, Chuck left the facility and found himself standing outside. He told me later he had the thought: "I don't want to be out here. It's raining!" That was the last incident I recorded in my log. Hallucinations and delusions often occur in the early stages of LBD and then cease.[49] *— Florrie Munat*

Florrie and Chuck were among the fortunate few. After a year, his behavioral symptoms stopped for some reason, although by then he had other symptoms.

Ted is in a new nursing home and on hospice. He's no longer able to get out of bed, and we can barely understand him when he tries to talk. Even so, the delusions and hallucinations still come around. — Jean

Ted's case, where the symptoms continued to the end, is a much more common occurrence.

Hallucinations can be due to a variety of disorders, including Parkinson's. The presence of Lewy body-related symptoms such as Active Dreams along with PD predicts eventual dementia. When hallucinations show up without PD, the accompaniment of other Lewy body symptoms also predicts the eventual presence of dementia with Lewy bodies (DLB), the type of LBD that occurs without PD.

While early hallucinations are defining symptoms of LBD, delusions and irrational anger are not--they also occur with too many other disorders. Even with other more unique LBD symptoms, such as Active Dreams, they can only be used to reinforce an already probable diagnosis. Nevertheless, these issues are some of the first cognitive symptoms that may appear and must be dealt with.

Chapter 11

Hallucinations and Illusions

Hallucinations are seeing something that isn't really there. Although usually visual, other senses such as auditory or touch can be involved. The loss of smell is an early Parkinson's symptom. If a PwPD appears to be able to smell again—usually something unpleasant—and seizures have been ruled out, the odors are probably olfactory hallucinations. Early hallucinations may be quite benign, with the person's insight still intact enough that the person knows that what they see is not real. At a PD support group:

Fred: My little dog, Blackie, goes with me everywhere.

Joan: I don't see him. Did you leave him home today?

Fred: No, he's here. But he's a hallucination—I can see him but I know he isn't real.

Joan: Doesn't that bother you?

Fred: Not at all, he's company—and I don't have to feed him or clean up after him!

A PwPD who hallucinates has an 80% chance of advancing to dementia within three years.[50] Eventually, Fred may not be able to tell the difference between what's real and what's not. At first, he may be able to reason well enough to accept a trusted person's word that what he sees isn't actually there. Then, with more cognitive losses, that same person's explanation will conflict with Fred's own view and frustrate rather than help him.

The PwPD may not tell anyone that he is experiencing hallucinations. The fact may come out only if a Lewy-savvy doctor asks during an office visit. Because hallucinations are such a strong indication of impending dementia, it is a good idea for the care partner to ask occasionally if this is a symptom the PwLB is experiencing. If the team hasn't already started to take measures to decrease symptoms, it is definitely time to do so now.

Hallucinations tend to be more disturbing to family members than to the one experiencing the event. Care partners used to be encouraged to explain to their loved ones that the hallucinations were unreal and what they say was their disorder:

Whenever Mom sees little animals all over, I gently explain to her that I know she sees them but I don't and then I remind her that it is her LBD acting up again. This usually works and she doesn't say anything more about the animals. — Marge

This may work for Marge, but being unnecessarily reminded of one's disabilities can be hurtful—and often ineffective as well. Unless your loved one is upset, the best way to deal with hallucinations is to ignore them. If that is not possible, enter into his reality enough to keep the peace.

Larry gets upset if I don't walk around the fuzzy little animals that he sees. I ask him tell me where they are so I can be sure to avoid them. I've found that way is a lot easier than arguing with him or even ignoring him. — Doris

Doris entered Larry's reality enough to keep him from being stressed. But she didn't join the drama; she didn't talk to the "fuzzy animals" or play with them.

Hallucinations are usually benign. However post-traumatic stress can make the episodes scary and stressful. People with war injuries, serious accidents, and other negative life events may find their past experiences showing up in their hallucinations and dreams. Exciting stimuli, such as a detective show or a thrilling adventure show on TV can do the same thing.

Illusions occur when a person sees something real as something else. Like hallucinations, these are common with LBD and can begin early on. Unlike hallucinations, they are not considered defining symptoms—they appear in too many other situations as well.

> *When Annie's dementia was still very mild, we flew to Europe. On the plane, she became alarmed when she saw a flickering overhead video monitor and believed it was a fire. I explained what it really was and she calmed down. Months later, Annie had a different response. When she saw a flickering light in a neighbor's window, I wasn't able to calm her until I distracted her attention with an ice cream cone.*
> *— Jim Whitworth*

Annie's LBD had progressed to where her loss of reasoning made it difficult for her to accept Jim's explanations. However, her decreased ability to focus made it easy for Jim to distract her. Both hallucinations and illusions can combine with delusional thinking.

Differences in hallucinations between disorders:

Hallucinations are common with Lewy body dementia, Alzheimer's and schizophrenia, but there are differences:

Onset:

AD: Hallucinations seldom appear until later stages.

LBD: Hallucinations often appear before cognitive symptoms.

Voices:

Schizophrenia: Hallucinations are usually "voices," often with demands for action.

LBD: Hallucinations are less likely to be audio and when they do appear, they are more often sounds such as a phone ringing rather than voices.

Chapter 12

Delusions

A delusion is a false, often paranoid belief, not subject to reason. Delusions are one of those symptoms that often accompany LBD although they cannot be identified as part of the dementia or MCI criteria. They are too common with so many other disorders. Nevertheless, they are often part of the disorder and cause enough concern to Lewy teams to earn inclusion here.

We were traveling and Gladys was driving. I became absolutely sure that she had taken us hundreds of miles off course. When she refused to turn around, I was frantic. I just knew that if she kept going, we'd be lost—if we weren't already. She told me to calm down, that she knew where we were and kept driving. I'm not a violent person but I really wanted to grab the wheel and make her stop. I don't know how I kept from doing that but I didn't. And then we got to familiar country and I relaxed. The next day I apologized to Gladys. Looking back, I know she was right. But I just couldn't get my mind around that at the time. — Clark

Clark was having a delusion. When he was feeling better, he remembered the event and was able to see his mistake. As the disorder advances, he probably won't be able to remember the event, or if he does, will still be stuck in his delusion. That's why this symptom is difficult to identify in oneself. Part of the delusion is that you truly believe your behavior is rational. Therefore, this chapter is directed mostly to the care partner or the person who will be on the receiving end of the delusional behavior rather than the person with the delusions.

The likelihood of delusions increases with age and with the presence of other risk factors, as all LBD symptoms do. Over 65% of all PwPD age 60 or older will experience delusions.[51] Some may find that the delusions are due to medication and that they will stop when the drugs are changed. However, this too should be viewed as a warning of eventual dementia—it's just a little bit further into the future.

Delusions can be triggered by many things besides drugs: pain, discomfort, feelings, memories, hallucinations, illusions, dreams, real events, or any combination thereof. The presence of delusions means that one's thinking skills are diminished although memory and other cognitive skills may be still be intact. The person may be able to understand a joke, remember birthdays or drive. However, his thinking filter, i.e., the ability to make judgments and control impulses, is damaged and thought processing steps get lost.

Here's a breakdown of how two people, one with and one without a well-functioning thinking filter, might view a similar event:

Brian, who does not have LBD, saw a flashing light in his neighbor's window. His first impression was that it looked a little like a fire and he felt a pang of fear. He looked closer and saw that it was a flickering TV screen. Then he laughed and walked on.

Annie, who does have LBD, saw a fire in her neighbor's window and screamed hysterically. Her husband, Jim, tried to tell her it was the neighbor's TV, but she continued to scream. Jim distracted her by pointing to a person coming towards them and asking her if it was someone they knew. She calmed down.

If we break the two stories down, they look like this:

The initial perception:

Both Brian and Annie see a flickering light in their neighbor's window and fear that it is a fire.

Applying the thinking filter:

Brian withholds judgment and takes a better look.

Annie ignores Jim's explanation and goes directly from fearing that the light is a fire to believing that it is a fire.

The final decision:

Brian decides the light is a flickering TV.

Annie accepts her first impression—the light *is a fire.*

The final feeling:

Brian feels relief.

Annie feels fear and helplessness.

The final response

Brian relaxes, laughs, and walks on.

Annie starts screaming hysterically and calms down only when she is distracted.

This whole sequence happens in just a moment or so. Brian felt some fear when he first saw the light in the window but he was able to use his thinking filter to gather more information and make a better judgment, which left him feeling positive and unstressed. With a faulty thinking filter, Annie could not think clearly enough to accept Jim's logical interpretation and was stuck with her feeling-based conclusions. She felt fear and helplessness, which led to her acting-out behavior.

> *Acting-out:* An apparently irrational, usually impulsive, and often difficult to control response to a real or imaginary stimulus.
>
> *A better definition*: A form of communication, usually stress related.

Annie believed that her neighbor's house was on fire—and no one was doing anything about it. No wonder she screamed! Her stimulus was the sight of what she labeled inaccurately as a fire (an illusion). For others, it might be a crowded room (real event), the false belief that one's care partner is poisoning them (a delusion) seeing a person that isn't really present (a hallucination) or an infection (pain and discomfort). Apparently irrational, the response feels quite rational to the person doing the acting-out, given his view of the situation.

Delusions that appear before other cognitive issues are noticed may unknowingly be treated as something other than the signs of a progressive disorder needing family, friend and co-worker support. Such treatment will increase stress and speed the progress of the disorder.

Right after Ralph turned 50 one of his co-workers asked me if something was wrong because he wasn't the even-tempered guy he used to be. He got in trouble at work because he was

yelling at coworkers and worse yet, the customers. Ralph's boss told him to shape up or he would be fired. Ralph tried, he really did. But the harder he tried, the more out of control he got. The boss made good on his promise and my husband was unemployed at 50—with little hope of finding another job. Thank goodness, I have a good job! Not long after that, Ralph ran a stop sign and caused a minor accident. That was the last straw. I insisted he see a doctor. I just knew there must be something wrong. The neurologist that the doctor referred him to diagnosed early dementia with Lewy bodies (DLB).
— Alix

Ralph had the kind of Lewy body disorder that can start with behavior problems instead of motor difficulties. Although Ralph's memory was still fair, the delusional behavior was evidence that his thinking abilities were affected. The pressure from Ralph's boss to change what he couldn't change only increased the delusions and the resulting behavior.

If Ralph had had Parkinson's disease, he, his family or his physician might have suspected PDD. However, Ralph was one of the 50% of LBD sufferers who skipped PD's motor symptoms and went directly to dementia symptoms.

DLB's early behavioral symptoms are more difficult to identify as Lewy-related than when the same symptoms appear in someone with PD. Therefore, Ralph went undiagnosed until his auto accident drove him to a physician. If he had received his diagnosis while he was still working, it could have led to more understanding and treatment that might have decreased his behavior or at least allowed for a medical retirement. Because such behaviors in a person who is young enough to still be employed are seldom connected with a degenerative disorder, let alone dementia, Ralph's situation is more common than one might think.

> **Warning:** When person's behavior changes drastically, family members should insist upon a referral to a neurologist—one who recognizes that behaviors sometime precede noticeable cognitive symptoms.

Delusions of spousal infidelity are especially common and, like other delusions, may start well before any other cognitive symptoms are noticeable. These can cause major emotional trauma for all family members concerned.

Ben retired last year. He's always been so invested in his work. He was still trying to adjust to being retired when he was diagnosed with MCI-LB. It's very mild—Ben still drives and reads the newspaper but it was a double whammy for him, for both of us, really—the retirement and then the diagnosis. He plays golf but says it isn't so much fun now that his scores aren't what they used to be. Still, I thought we were doing all right until last month, when he started accusing me of meeting other men. A half-hour trip to the grocery store is a tryst with my lover. A chat on the phone with my daughter is phone sex. The more I explain that I'd never do any of that, the worse Ben gets. I'm at my wits end! — Marjorie

Unlike Clark, Ben doesn't see later on that his behavior was delusional. This is much more common. The more intense the fear, the stronger the delusion. Ben's retirement and diagnosis, with its accompanying losses, like worse golf scores, brought about strong feelings of inadequacy. He fears that Marjorie would no longer view him as a desirable companion. With LBD weakening his thinking filters, Ben accepts what he *fears* as *fact*. Thus in Ben's mind, Marjorie *is* deserting him. This is terrifying to Ben. If Marjorie leaves him, how will he cope? Ben's anger is his effort to communicate his fears of abandonment.

Several things impact Ben's behavior:

Ben's delusion: His damaged thinking filter impairs judgment and turns his fear that Marjorie will leave him into "fact."

> *Fix:* Start with a healthy, active, low stress lifestyle to keep thinking abilities functional as long as possible. Dementia drugs may improve thinking filters and reduce delusions, even early in the journey before other cognitive losses are noticeable.

The intensity of Ben's feelings: The stronger the fear, the stronger the belief. To Ben, they are one and the same.

> *Fix:* Decrease the fear by maintaining a loving and caring attitude.

> *Fix:* Talk about past experiences that were very positive—vacations you had and other such mutually enjoyable times. This may not be effective during the delusion—it needs to be an ongoing activity.

Marjorie's denial: Ben perceives Marjorie's denial of his "facts" as a denial of his emotions—which leaves him feeling even more deserted.

Fix: Talk about the feelings, not the facts—real or imagined, and try to say something that implies that you are in this together. Support the feelings instead of denying the accusation. Marjorie might say something like, "A lot has been going on. I can understand how you'd be worried. It's a lot to handle for both of us."

The intensity of Marjorie's denial: When Marjorie shows her frustrations and hurt at being accused falsely, Ben mirrors the intensity of those feelings with increased negative feelings of his own—and an increased belief in his delusion.

Fix: Stay calm and avoid expressing negative feelings. Marjorie can calmly say something non-committal such as, "I'm right here and I'm not leaving" and then change the subject. (In this case, another symptom becomes helpful—attention deficit prevents Ben from maintaining focus for very long and makes it easier to distract him onto another subject.)

Fix: Take a break. If Marjorie feels herself getting caught up in the argument, she can leave for a few minutes, take several deep breaths and remind herself "It's the disorder." This will help her maintain the distance needed to keep her calm.

Disagreement between Marjorie's words and her body language: When Marjorie tells Ben she loves him but her body language shows her natural frustration, Ben will believe her non-verbal message and discount her words.

Fix: Be aware of non-verbal communication. Marjorie must make sure that her tone and actions are gentle and caring, not sharp and angry.

Ben's fixation on the subject. When Ben feels his message isn't receiving adequate attention, he will continue with his behavior.

Fix: Respond to feelings, which are real, rather than his "facts" which are garbled.

Fix: If words don't help, distract by changing the subject. Marjorie might offer a snack or even a ride in the car.

If these solutions don't work, Ben's doctor may suggest a behavior management drug. Of course, the drug must be monitored carefully. If the acting-out becomes dangerous and can't be controlled, residential care may need to be considered.

Harry believes that the neighbor's dog is our old, long dead dog, Hambone. That the dog now lives next door seems not to bother Harry. Once I learned not to try to correct Harry's misbelief, and just let him enjoy the dog when he comes to visit, I did fine too. –Lydia

Delusions may also be benign, or not stressful, as with Harry and Hambone. Like hallucinations, they can be more stressful for care partners until, like Lydia, they learn to accept, and ignore or work around the delusion enough to pacify their loved one.

Care partners report that with the progression of the disorder, delusions become less and may eventually stop especially when the dementia gets more severe. Delusions require a certain amount of thinking ability, even if it is irrational.

Intensity: The intensity of a feeling and its positive or negative charge is more important than words. Thus a frustrated "But I do love you" is heard as a denial of love. Calmness draws out calmer responses.

The value of positives: It takes about five positives to counteract one negative, more if the negative is a delusion. Therefore, loving behavior needs to be continual and ongoing, even exaggerated as long as the feeling is real.

Harmony: As thinking abilities decrease, the awareness of feelings and body language increase. These must be in harmony with your words or what you say will be rejected.

Reality vs. belief: As thinking ability disappears, reality becomes less important than belief. That isn't going to change. Reminding a person of their loss is painful and unnecessary.

Chapter 13

Fluctuating Abilities and Symptoms

The literature usually refers to this Lewy body symptom as "fluctuating cognition." However, other abilities also vary. These fluctuations can start early, even before MCI is recognized. For instance, PwPD are probably already aware that sometimes they have better motor control than at other times— that their ability to move changes with what may seem to be very little reason. A variety of other LB symptoms, such as hallucinations and delusions, may also come and go.

Thinking ability, attention and alertness can fluctuate from week to week, day to day, minute to minute. Early hallucinations or delusions will usually come in short episodes and then may not show up again for quite a while—long enough to fool many people into thinking they won't ever show up again. These fluctuations tend to affect many abilities at the same time: For instance, confusion may accompany behavioral symptoms and there could be motor problems as well.

PwLB may occasionally be able to remember their episodes of confusion as Clark did in Chapter 12. However, the more common experience is no memory, or at the most, partial memory of the event. There is often a pattern, however. For instance, a person is likely to do better when rested or unstressed.

The presence of fluctuating symptoms is relatively unique to LBD, thus helpful with a diagnosis. For example, early delusions are symptoms of both LBD and Frontotemporal Dementia

(FTD), which is actually more common if the person is middle-aged. If the delusions come and go, LBD might be suspected but if they are continuous, then FTD is more likely.

Care partners call the periods of high and low functioning the Good Times and Bad Times. They say that living with LBD is like riding a roller coaster, with continual ups and downs. When Good Times are the norm, as they often are in MCI, an unexpected delusional episode can be quite frightening.

Al began having delusions and accused me of stealing his money. When he got physical, I became frightened and called his doctor who admitted him to a hospital. I liked the doctor and she seemed to know about LBD—she was really careful about the drugs. He was only there a few days when his delusions stopped and he was discharged. I was ecstatic! Al was so much better—why, we even uh, made love the night he came home. That's not happened for so long it's a wonder I remembered how! And then, Al was delusional again. This time he thought I was a nurse in bed with him—but still after his money. I was devastated. I thought he was well. But now, he's just as bad as he ever was—No, he's worse. He didn't even know me! — Florence

Fluctuations make it easy to think that the delusional episode was just a bad spell, like a case of the flu that comes and, when it has run its course, leaves forever. Florence definitely did the right thing when she called the doctor. Especially if there is a threat of violence, you should not try to deal with an irrational person by yourself, at least until you know how to do so.

However, these "spells" return. The usual pattern is that at first, the LB symptom appears for only a short time with long intervals between events. The length of the episodes gets longer and the time between them gets shorter, until that behavior becomes the norm. Then you will see episodes of more alert behavior, which conversely, get shorter and further apart.

As Florence learns to expect these changes as a part of Al's disorder, she won't be so devastated when they occur. However, they can still be disheartening even for the more seasoned care partner.

> *I know that Aaron's condition fluctuates and for the most part, I've accepted it and roll with it. But when his Good Times last for several days, it is so easy to forget that they are temporary. Instead of enjoying our normalness for the respite that it is, I slip back into the old comfort of being a part of a couple instead of a caregiver. Then when LBD symptoms come back—and they always do—I experience the same sense of desertion and loneliness I felt when he first disappeared into his confusion. I have to work through to acceptance all over again. You'd think I'd learn, but somehow, I don't—I'm riding that rollercoaster right along with Aaron. — Jeanette*

For many care partners, acceptance is not a one-time task. As the norm changes from alertness to confusion, care partners do learn to adjust. Like Jeanette, they accept that their life has changed. The care partners enjoy flashes of awareness from their loved ones as temporary and limited. However, longer periods of awareness can be both more enjoyable and more difficult. The care partner finds it all too easy to be lulled into a false security, inevitably followed by a rude awakening when their rollercoaster heads back down into confusion. Then the work of acceptance must be done again. Understanding the dynamics of LBD keeps that effort from being as difficult as it originally was.

The care partner's job changes with the fluctuations. During the Bad times, the PwLBD needs more help but during Good times, this help may seem intrusive and degrading.

Some days Ken is on top of everything and he lets me know that I am really being bossy. I have to rethink the situation and realize that he is having a good day and doesn't need my help. It's embarrassing when he tells me off in front of others. I've learned to just shrug my shoulders—but I've also learned to stop and take the time to judge Ken's abilities before I barge right in with help. — Kathy

LBD's unique fluctuations can cause other problems. A physician who doesn't understand this symptom can impair a family's efforts to obtain the help they need from the Veteran Affairs (VA), insurance companies and the like.

While Al was in the hospital, the social worker told us about the VA Long Term Care benefits. I was so relieved; I'd been worrying about how we were going to pay for residential care if Al needed it. We applied immediately and just before Al was discharged, they told me that our application was only one signature away from being accepted. When Al got worse again, I was afraid to keep him at home any longer. I called the VA and that's when I learned that he was no longer eligible for these benefits—according to his hospital records, he had "recovered" and didn't qualify anymore. I had to reapply. — Florence

This is another example of why LB families need to stay informed even when their physician appears to be Lewy-savvy. Sometimes, like Al's doctor, the medical staff may be aware of the really dangerous issues such as drugs but aren't as informed about symptoms like fluctuating cognition. Or the doctor may know but isn't careful to write discharges and conditions in a way that reflects LBD's cycle of repeated ups and downs. Then equally unaware agencies approve or disapprove applications for care, based on what the physician writes.

> *Carl would shuffle into the doctor's reception lobby. Then as we went back to the office, my husband would straighten up and actually walk down the hall. Carl doesn't talk much anymore but he was saying whole sentences to the doctor. Why can't he do that with me? -- Megan*

Carl was experiencing "Showtime," a type of fluctuation where the PwLBD functions better in the presence of someone other than the care partner. This is not something he can control. It tends to happen at times when a person would normally want to make a good impression, such as at the doctor's office or with visiting adult children. If a doctor or family member is not Lewy-savvy, he or she may believe what he sees rather than a care partner's report. Showtime can last from a few minutes to a day or so. It uses up a lot of energy and therefore, is usually followed by extreme tiredness.

Sometimes what looks like a typical Lewy body fluctuation is actually drug related. When a person acts out in response to LBD symptoms such as delusions, many non-Lewy-savvy nurses or doctors will increase or add medication. That may make the problem worse. Then, when the drugs are withdrawn, there may be radical improvement. This does not mean recovery; LBD is still there. Without the irritation of the inappropriate or excessive drugs, it has simply calmed down—for a while. A Lewy-savvy doctor is important, but you still need to keep informed. With fluctuations, no matter what their cause, it is probably more important to have a doctor who will listen than to have a Lewy-savvy doctor.

> ***Showtime:*** A period of better functioning that is NOT under the PwLBD's control, usually followed by lower than normal functioning and extended sleeping. Use a daily journal to help family or physicians know about the everyday issues that may not appear during Showtime.

LBD is unpredictable. Its symptoms can appear together or alone. Symptoms may fluctuate or leave with as little warning as when they first appeared. Usually, other symptoms will take their place.

Just when I became used to Kevin's hallucinations, everything changed,. He quit hallucinating and started having problems with swallowing. I dread to think what will be next! — Sarah

Like any progressive disorder, the PwLB's condition on the average will continually go downhill. The fluctuations will be a little lower and will seldom return to the previous high. This can continue for years. However, LBD is also known for its sudden, deep downturns of functioning.

Del was doing well in Assisted Living and then one day, I came in and he was far more confused than he had been. He wasn't as mobile either. He was agitated and irritable—he was just so much worse. The staff and I tried to figure out what was different but we couldn't identify anything. No medication changes, nothing. He tended to have UTIs and so I asked that they check for that and sure enough, he had one. They took care of that, but Del just never came back to anywhere near as good as he'd been. He died about six months later. — Nancy

These sudden slides usually occur well into the LB journey unless they are caused by stress from illnesses, surgery or inappropriate drugs. As the disorder progresses, the PwLBD's ability to deal with stress decreases and major downturns become harder to prevent. Del's reaction to a reoccurring urinary tract infection was an example of this. He had been gradually getting worse, losing abilities and being more confused. Nancy found she could no longer care for him and so he was in Assisted Living. He had weathered many UTIs, but this one sent him into a slide from which he never recovered.

Section Two:

Taking Control

People tend to act one of two ways when faced with a life-changing diagnosis. The first is to ignore it and stay stuck in denial.

> *I'm fine. I'm just a little forgetful. At my age, that's expected.* — *Annie*

> *I have PD. Isn't that enough for us to deal with? Now we have to think about dementia too? No, thank you, I'd rather deal with it when the time comes—if it ever does.* — *Edwin*

Annie didn't have a problem and she didn't want to know anything about this problem she "didn't have." Edwin's attitude is understandable too. Knowing that dementia is in your future can be too frightening to consider. Neither he nor Annie could understand that hiding can make it even more frightening.

The second way of responding to a life changing diagnosis is to accept it and move on.

> *It took a while but eventually, we realized that we couldn't change the fact that Del's Parkinson's had progressed and now he had PDD. But we could control how we dealt with it. We educated ourselves and learned to adapt.* — *Nancy*

Nancy and Del believed that knowledge was power and wanted to know everything possible about what they were dealing with.

This book is for people like Nancy and Del, for people who want to be armed with all the information they can find.

Everyone wants to be in control of their lives. Lewy body dementia is a thief that slowly steals away the ability to do that-- from the PwLBD and from the family as well. When a person receives a LBD diagnosis, life as they and their family knew it will never be the same. Not necessarily worse, at least not right away, but definitely different. Anyone dealing with LBD must learn new ways of thinking, acting and living. This is not an option; it is a requirement of the disorder.

Experiencing a difficult situation is much like going through the grief process. In fact, people do experience this process when dealing with any progressively degenerative disorder. It is normal to feel the denial the Edwin and Annie felt. No one wants to know that their life isn't going as expected; that may take over and make unacceptable changes. It is normal to feel anger as well.

However, the Lewy team doesn't have to stay stuck in any of these painful feelings. It takes work and even faith, but it is possible to move on and reach acceptance. Learning to adapt rather than deny offers a feeling of power and control. The more you can take charge, the easier this journey will be for the whole family.

Chapter 14

Getting the Right Diagnosis

Often the first step towards taking control is getting a diagnosis.

> *I knew something was wrong for years before I could convince my primary doctor to send me to a neurologist. Maybe it was my age. I was in my 50's. I'd make mistakes at home and my wife would just laugh and take over the job. I'd mess up at work and my coworkers would excuse it with "we all make mistakes now and then." No one wanted to think that it might be dementia. No one wanted to say the "d" word.[52] — Rick Phelps*

Rick had early onset Alzheimer's. However, it is even more common for people with LBD to be the first to notice that something is wrong. Their executive losses (organization, multitasking, etc), aren't so evident to doctors and family. Many will be older than Rick but still, the symptoms will likely be present long before a doctor recognizes a problem. The path to diagnosis can be difficult for the person with MCI or with early onset dementia. As with Rick, no one wants to admit there is a problem. The final push to diagnosis may come after a crisis such as an auto accident, work disruption or an embarrassing confrontation.

Even then, family and friends may find it difficult to accept the changes. Although PwLB may also fight acceptance, many are glad to discover an organic reason for their loss of functioning.

The next step is to persevere until there is a diagnosis that fits the symptoms. With LBD, the first one often does not. It is common for a person to see several doctors and receive three or more diagnoses before getting one for LBD. Usually something else, such as Alzheimer's or PD is diagnosed first.[53] Diagnosis can be a long arduous process covering years and multiple guesses, often partly right but not addressing all the symptoms. Maybe there is Parkinson's, or even Alzheimer's, but there's more that remains unexplained. Even when Lewy body dementia is finally diagnosed, the discoveries don't end. LBD is a disorder of change. The PwLBD will repeatedly find old ways of doing things no longer work. It is an ongoing process.

Anyone dealing with Lewy body disorders soon discovers that the varied aspects and symptoms require a team of professionals. The PwLBD may start out with just a primary physician and a movement specialist, but as the disorder advances, others, such as a dementia specialist, an internist and a variety of therapists may join the team.

Choosing a specialist. The *Guide* has a chapter on choosing specialists (page 13) and another on building a health care team (page 169). As time goes on, the care partner becomes a specialist on the way the PwLBD expresses this changeable disorder simply from living with it daily. Add some research and that knowledge may seem to equal that of the doctor's—in just that single area, of course.

> *I sometimes feel that Jacob's neurologist should be paying me. She admits that she hasn't had many LBD patients and is continually asking me questions about what I've researched or what I've learned from working with Jacob. Even so, I feel better with her than with someone who wouldn't listen to me.* —Betty

Betty's neurologist understands that care partners are often well informed about this disorder and she is willing to listen and learn. Good treatment is a cooperative experience. The doctors need the Lewy team's input for an accurate evaluation of the disorder's progress. The team needs the specialists for their greater expertise and the primary physician to keep track of the whole picture.

With this in mind, choose physicians who recognize the care partner as a part of the treatment team and don't brush you off with "I know best" type of responses. Ideally the doctors are Lewy-savvy. Doctors who listen, and then use their own expertise to put your information to use, are almost as good.

The diagnostic process. The normal process is that you will first see a primary doctor who will refer you to a specialist, usually a neurologist. You might also be referred to a psychiatrist. Geriatric psychiatrists (those specializing in the elderly) are usually safe. Others may be too—if they are Lewy-savvy. However, caregivers have found that many psychiatrists prefer Lewy-sensitive drugs for behavior and anxiety management. If you are already dealing with PD, your neurologist is likely a movement specialist. Ask what they know about LBD and its sensitivities to drugs, including some PD drugs. Many movement specialists are now well informed about these issues. However, if yours does not appear to be, ask for a referral to a dementia specialist.

Either the primary doctor or the specialist or both will likely administer some tests and then tell you their opinion. An accurate diagnosis depends more on the doctor's ability to recognize a Lewy body disorder than it does on the accuracy of the tests. As yet, there is no objective test that confirms the presence of any LB disorder—or any other neurological disorder, for that matter.

A second opinion. If the symptoms and the diagnosis don't match, ask for a second opinion. Some doctors will say that the name of the dementia doesn't matter. With LBD and its drug sensitivity issues, the name does. If there is even a chance that a person has this type of dementia, the medical community needs to know.

With the proper diagnosis and ICD-9 (International Classification of Diseases, 9th revision) insurance codes, physicians can treat LBD's unique symptoms appropriately. Having a diagnosis of Lewy body dementia, dementia with Lewy bodies, or Parkinson's disease with dementia or something similar to these in a person's chart will alert the medical community to avoid Lewy-sensitive drugs.

People who have gone through a complete evaluation often balk at doing memory quizzes, drawing things, or other such assessments again. It is demoralizing to take tests that show how much one's mental capacity has declined. If the tests are too painful, the Lewy team can ask that no new ones be administered once a formal diagnosis of any type of LBD has been made. However, the new tests can provide insights regarding presence of other issues that may need treatment and so the team may want to allow them.

Diagnostic Tests

These tests require special equipment and are usually only done in larger research or teaching centers.

The Single Photon Emission Computed Tomography (SPECT) scan test.[54] This combination of computed tomography (CT) scan and an injected radioisotope produces a 3-D image of the brain. It can be helpful for identifying even early LBD. The administration process requires special training. While CT scans are available in most hospitals, radioisotopes have a short life and are therefore only available where they are manufactured, i.e., in large medical centers.

Dopamine Transporter (DaT) scan.[55] This is a SPECT scan using a radioactive drug that binds to dopamine transporters in the brain. Experts consider it more effective in differentiating LBD from AD than other SPECT scans.

Heart imaging. A radioactive tracer used with heart imaging that is called ^{123}I-metaiodobenzylguanidine (MIBG),[56] can make a distinction between the Lewy body disorders and AD. It has even been known to correctly predict LBD in people who had amnestic MCI (the type that usually precedes AD).

These tests can be done in a primary physician's office.

The Mini-Mental State Exam (MMSE).[57] This mini-exam has been in use for a long time and takes only a few minutes in your doctor's office. It has a good record of identifying dementia in general. It is often combined with the SPECT test for good results in identifying probable LBD.

A battery of tests that improve the MMSE's ability to identify LBD even at early stages:[58]

- The MMSE, given and scored with an emphasis on orientation.
- The clock drawing test, where the person being tested draws a clock with a designated time showing.
- The cube drawing test, where the person copies a 3-D picture of a cube.

The Montreal Cognitive Assessment (MoCA).[59] This screening tool developed in 2010 takes about ten minutes to administer. It assesses the domains of attention and concentration, executive functions, memory, language, visuospatial skills, conceptual thinking, calculations, and orientation. More sensitive than the above MMSE and better at identifying non-memory impairments, this tool is can be used without additional tests such as the clock drawing and is becoming the test of choice.

After the Diagnosis

Once there is a diagnosis, you and your loved one will likely have many confusions and questions that few doctors have the time to answer.

> *Ted's neurologist spent 20 minutes explaining what LBD was but we were too shell-shocked to ask any questions. When we got home, we couldn't remember much of what he said. The good part was that he had us make an appointment with a nurse-counselor. We had dozens of questions and concerns for her. She was wonderful. She answered all our questions and gave us a list of places we could go for added support. She*

even showed us some websites that were especially helpful. —
Jean

If your Lewy team is fortunate, the neurologist will do as Ted's did and send you to someone who has plenty of time for questions and concerns. If the doctor doesn't do this, ask for a referral. If that isn't available, ask about support groups.

If there is a local LBD caregiver support group in the area, contact it and go with a support person. Loved ones may or may not be able to attend. Also contact local organizations such as the Area Agency on Aging, or even the closest Senior Center. LBD people report mixed experiences with Alzheimer's or Parkinson's support groups because the focus is not quite the same as it is with a LBD group. Even so, these groups are worth trying. See the Resource Section for more suggestions for help and support.

Chapter 15

The Grieving Process

You might not think that grieving is a part of taking control. Some do refuse to grieve, or rather refuse to recognize that they are grieving. These people give up the chance of moving on to a place where taking control is possible. When you recognize the possibility that a degenerative disorder is in your future, there will be grief. You grieve for the life your Lewy team expected and can no longer hope to have. You grieve for the things you may no longer be able to do. This will be an ongoing process, sometimes more severe than others.

Grief about a degenerative disorder like Parkinson's or LBD is a seven-step process.[60]

Shock. This initial paralysis blocks feeling and allows time to recover and move on. Shock is usually very short lived—only an hour, or a day or so.

Denial. You begin to have feelings again, but block out the possibility of the disorder. You resist the suggestion that LBD may be in your future. *Surely they are wrong. I can't have this. We can't have this.*

Denial is a normal, even healthy reaction when the first warning signs of LBD are noticed, or even when that first diagnosis is received. It blocks out the pain of such an unwanted life change and gives you time to adjust. It is nature's way of letting in only as much as you can handle. Some people stay in this step and never leave it. Family members who aren't living with the disorder day by day may be unable to move past denial.

When denial lasts past the adjustment period it becomes destructive. It blocks you from taking control and doing anything to deal with the problem. Worse, it is never completely effective. When denial fails, the pain of what you perceive as an unbearable truth drives you into an even deeper denial. All of this adds stress which will make what you are avoiding (Lewy) even more ferocious, and therefore more difficult to avoid.

Anger. Feeling anger gives you strength to face this difficult life event and energy to move on. You are beginning to accept the reality of the diagnosis and you rail against it. *Why me? Why us?* For people who don't consider anger an acceptable feeling, this can be the most difficult part of the grieving. *How can I feel angry at God? At my partner? Why am I angry all the time? I used to be a very nice person and now I'm a shrew.* Anger is a natural part of the grief process. Repressing or bottling up the anger inside will only make you feel worse. The more you let yourself express it, the sooner it will pass.

Anger is another step that family members may get stuck in. Expressing disapproval and anger at the way someone else is handling their loved one's situation may be their way of participating—not a very helpful way, but fairly common.

Bargaining. You are seeking in vain for a way out. *OK, I believe the diagnosis but there must be something I can do, we can do, something someone can do to change it, to bring back the life we had.*

Guilt is a close companion of bargaining. It is an effort to control the past. *If only I'd...We should have...Why didn't I...* are all useless recriminations about the past. What is, is. Guilt just adds stress to an already stressful situation.

Depression. The final realization of the inevitable. Yes, the diagnosis is true. *Our lives are over, done. Why bother?* This situational depression is a natural *short-term* response to any loss and this is definitely a serious, ongoing loss. However, depression is also a LB disorder symptom. When the PwLB's depression lasts a long time, it may need to be treated. There are some medications for chronic depression that are less Lewy-sensitive.

Testing. As you stop being so depressed, you become interested in looking for more realistic answers. OK, this is the life we have. *What can we do, what can I do, to make it better, tolerable, more enjoyable?*

Acceptance. You begin to find meaning in the life you have, not the one you wish you had. This acceptance allows you to release the energy and power once used for avoidance, anger, guilt or self-pity and use it to move on, to take advantage of the testing you did. *Life is still worth living. I can do this.* Take a breath, relax a little.

As humans, we cycle through these steps more than once, often changing the order, skipping one, feeling stuck in another. You may be angry and then accepting, and then in denial and then feeling guilty, and then angry again. Just knowing that it is a natural process will get you through it more easily, although perhaps "easily" is not the right word. Grieving is never easy, but it *is* necessary.

The alternative is to be stuck in one of the steps with unacknowledged feelings lurking around and blindsiding you at unexpected moments. Accepting and allowing yourself to experience these painful feelings makes them less powerful and easier to release. Then you can move on.

Because LB disorders are progressive, anyone involved with them will continually be dealing with new losses and new feelings to process. However, as you learn the process, it will take less time and you will be able to stay in acceptance longer.

Grieving is an individual process. Everyone goes at their own speed. The PwLBD may or may not be able to make these changes along with you. He may need your help to let go of now unrealistic expectations and move to a more accepting place. Or you may need his. Be patient. It will happen.

Chapter 16

Choosing Acceptance

Working through the grief cycle and making a conscious choice to accept this new future allows you to feel more in control of your life. Not that choosing acceptance is easy, or even that it is a one-time event. You will have to do it over and over, daily perhaps.

Accepting early symptoms as warning signals opens you up to learning how to extend the PwLB's awareness and limit confusion. Accepting the diagnosis allows your team to learn ways to work around it and adapt. It is a scientific fact that acting with intent makes one happier and healthier. This is true even when dealing with a progressive disorder like LBD. Acting with intent provides a feeling of power and makes the disorder feel more manageable.

My cat, Panther, was king of our home—until my grown daughter came to visit with her two small dogs. Panther hid from the noisy, bothersome creatures for two days. When he showed his face, the dogs were there, chasing him back into hiding. On the third day, he stalked out into the living room. Of course, the dogs ran after him at full voice. But Panther had had enough. He stood his ground. One dog yelped when he got close enough to feel the cat's claw. Both dogs turned tail. After that, Panther had the run of the house again. The dogs were still noisy and bothersome, but he'd learned he could make them back off. – Helen Whitworth

LBD is like this. It is scary and you may feel compelled to spend all your energy and resources hiding from it and protecting yourself from its unwelcome invasion. This allows the disorder to do just what you fear. It takes over your life, limiting it much sooner and much more than need be. You have to be like Panther, willing to accept what is and stand your ground.

Accepting is *not* giving up. It is not just settling. It is taking charge. Accept *what is* and make that your base, the reality of your life. From there, you can take charge and challenge the disorder's progress. Taking charge makes the truth more bearable. Not what you wanted, but definitely bearable.

By the way, taking charge does not mean that you take charge of your loved one and run his life. It means that you take charge of your life and make it more livable. As the PwLB develops his own feelings of acceptance, he will also have a feeling of being more in control of his life. Because the degenerative nature of LB disorders gradually makes feeling in control of one's own body more and more difficult, this is extremely important.

Making Changes

Taking charge is like developing any other habit. As you make these changes, your loved one will be able to mirror them. Here are a few suggestions that will help:

Accept again—and again. Because of the disorder's continually changing character, acceptance is seldom a one-time event. Just when you think you have accepted the disorder, it changes and there's more disability or a new symptom--and you must grieve and work through to acceptance all over again. Don't rush this. Just do the best you can do and move on.

Replace negatives with positives. You can't just stop being negative. Nature hates a vacuum; if you don't consciously choose a positive thought or feeling, the negatives will be replaced by other negatives. Take charge. As soon as you recognize a negative thought or feeling, replace it. When trying to let go of a bad habit, replace it with a good one.

Use rephrasing. Start with LBD. In the past the "D" stood for *Dementia.* This word often has bad connotations. However, LBD truly is a *Disorder*—a group of harmful symptoms. Yes, dementia is part of the disorder, but it is part of many disorders. Use *progressive* instead of *degenerative.* Both are true, but progressive reminds you that while LB disorders will progress, you can do much to decrease the severity of the symptoms. LBD is *treatable*, rather than *incurable.* True there is no cure, but there are many ways to treat it; to decrease its symptoms, or make it less damaging. Keep on the lookout for new words to rephrase. Each one helps.

Use humor. Choose laughter instead of embarrassment. When the PwLBD messes up doing something that used to be easy, joke about it. Laugh with, not at him, of course. Like denial, embarrassment is stressful and holds you back. Humor releases tension and allows you to move on. It may not be easy to laugh or joke about something that feels so frightening and serious at first, but it becomes easier as you make humor a part of your team's treatment.

Talk about it. The more openly you can talk about the disorder, the more comfortable you will become with it. This will help your loved one be more comfortable as well. When it is simply a fact of life to be worked around, it stops being a scary monster taking up so much emotional space. When you share what's going on with others, you will discover that they are more interested than rejecting, more supportive than pitying. This doesn't mean harping on it all the time—especially if the disorder is so advanced that PwLBD has little insight into his deficits. It simply means being open and willing to talk as needed.

Have realistic expectations. Yes, you need to have realistic expectations for your loved one and the disorder. However, don't forget yourself. A care partner isn't Superwoman/man! You *will* feel angry, lonely, frightened, frustrated, overwhelmed, tired, etc. Don't expect this to be an easy job. Be gentle with yourself and with your family.

Look for the challenge. Overcoming a challenge is uplifting but as one's body changes, these challenges may seem few and far between. That doesn't need to be. Opportunities for challenge abounds when the focus changes from improving abilities to keeping them. Encourage the PwLBD to set goals that make him work hard enough to feel good when he succeeds. There is a balance here. Goals that are too high are a setup for failure. As cognition slides, goals must change too or he will be overwhelmed.

My mom, Andrea, was really creative. Her scrapbooks are filled with great pictures and beautiful calligraphy. She quit the fancy writing when her tremors got too bad, but kept on scrapbooking. Then she stopped. "I can't do it anymore," she told me. When I asked her why, she just shook her head. I tried to get her to do a page. That's when I realized that her MCI had stolen her ability to plan—to figure out where to put what. She'd either just paste her pictures in anywhere, or hand the picture to me with "You do it." We still get out Mom's scrapbooks but now, it's a time for us to talk about what she did in the past. We open a book to a scene and she'll tell me about it—about the trip she took, the play she attended, etc. I challenge her to dig deeper into her memory for more about that time in her life—the people, the events, etc. It's become a time of sharing and we both love it. — Robyn

Robyn recognized that scrapbooking had moved from being a challenge to being an overwhelming and unrewarding activity. She changed it so that her mother could still enjoy her hobby and continue to be challenged by it in its new form. You can do the same. When an activity goes from being a challenge to a burden, change it to something that is still rewarding. That may be the hardest part—being willing to accept and move on.

As a team, be active adventurers instead of passive accepters of fate. This is not in conflict with having realistic expectations. Take charge, be optimistic, set goals and work to make it happen. Plan trips and projects. Make your objectives big enough to be challenging. Be willing to risk failure and try again.

Create a big dream instead of assuming the worst. Shoot for the moon and be willing to do whatever it takes to get there. Take reasonable risks and be willing to laugh when your plan doesn't work out.[61] — Judy Towne Jennings

Be brave. No one says that letting go of denial or making changes is easy. They both mean moving from the familiar to the uncharted, often the unwanted. Being brave does not mean that you stop being afraid or wary of what the future holds. Soldiers in battle are very fearful. Yet, they step up anyway and do their job. The two of you are soldiers in this battle. You can crouch in fear behind your denial or swallow, take a deep breath and move forward. Being afraid is also what keeps a soldier alert for problems. For you, it means checking facts and asking for second opinions. It means finding the right physician, specialists and other support people.

Become a seeker instead of an avoider. Make it your job to learn as much as you can about LB disorders. Find a support group; use the Internet to research; ask questions. As you put energy into knowing and understanding this disorder that has invaded your family, you will fear it less. The end result is a better quality of life.

Look for the joy. This doesn't have to be big. It can be enjoying a walk or a joke with your loved one, reading a book with a grandchild, eating a favorite food or succeeding at a challenging task. Stay alert for such pleasant events and celebrate each one.

> *Every once in a while the "old" Al appears. He will offer me a hug or tell a real joke. I save these times up to remember when I'm feeling sad, just like I do beautiful sunsets and the smell of full-blown roses. — Florence*

Every person and every family finds their own way to acceptance. Judy and her husband rephrased their LBD journey as an adventure. Florence saved up memories to help her coast over the blue times. Use the tips below to help as you find your own path.

One day at a time. Alcohol Anonymous uses this phrase well. Deal with only one day, one hour, one minute at a time to make it through rough spots more easily and enjoy positives more thoroughly. Make changes, one small thing at a time. With success, try another change. *Do not try to do everything at once.*

Have support. Family and friends are on this journey with you. They are affected too. Work together. Make it a cooperative venture. The lifestyle changes needed to keep LBD in check are good for everyone, not just for the person with the disorder. Reach out to your friends, church groups and others. Join a support group in your community, or online or both.

Keep a journal. LB disorders are very changeable. They are both progressive and fluctuating. Thus, what you see today may not be the same tomorrow, or next week. A journal helps to keep track of what you've been doing to stay in charge and make changes. Use it to keep track of goals, symptoms and medications along with their results. Combine your journal with a calendar to keep better track of activities. Finally, use it as a private place to vent. Every care partner needs this!

Chapter 17

Medical, Legal and Financial Choices

This whole area of choices and decisions needs to be addressed early in the LB journey. It starts with choosing doctors and other medical personnel who will support you as a team. It goes on to include all the legal and financial paperwork that makes it possible for the care partner to carry on when the PwLBD can no longer share in the decision making. It also includes planning for the expenses involved with any progressive disorder.

Medical Choices

Disorders such as LBD require a team of medical professionals, from primary care physician to neurologist to people like physical and speech therapists. In each case, make sure these people are

- As Lewy-savvy as possible and
- Willing to listen to the care partner.

The last condition is probably the most important. As the disorder advances, the care partner will often be the person who knows the most about their charge's particular symptoms. The PwLBD may not remember more difficult times—or may not see them as difficult. LBD plays tricks on doctors and often hides its true nature behind "Showtime," appearing much better than at home. (See Chapter 13, and the *Guide*, pg. 52) Therefore, it is mandatory that medical personnel include the care partner as a part of the treatment team. Make sure proper permissions are signed so that they can talk to you.

Planning For the Future

Lewy teams need to take some time early in the journey to make legal and financial decisions for the future. The earlier this is done, the more input the PwLB will be able to have. It is important for the care partner to do the same preparation. Care partners are at high risk for illness and even death. Naturally, the changes don't have to start now. They just need to be in place. Each partner should start by answering the following questions:

- Who do I want to manage funds, pay bills and make financial and legal decisions if I no longer can?
- Who do I want to make my medical decisions?
- Who can take the care partner's place, should that be needed?

Getting your wishes down in writing and out of the way is a great stress reliever. The authors made these decisions together in the first year of marriage while both were in good health. Don't wait for warning signs. Just get it done. Then you don't have to worry about it anymore. Well, that's not quite true. You should review all of your paperwork once a year or so and make sure everything is still what you want.

Use an Elder Care Attorney. Make sure your decisions hold up legally. Contact an attorney who is familiar with the needs of the elderly in general and dementia specifically. This person can explain what is needed to make a smooth transition for when the PwLBD can no longer make decisions or the care partner becomes ill. For a start, ask about the following:

Durable power of attorney. This document allows a chosen person to make decisions when the person no longer can. The attorney will likely recommend one for legal/financial matters and another for health care decisions.

A Living Will or Health Care Directive. This provides medical staff with the information they need to provide proper care. When a person identifies the type of medical care wanted, others don't have to second guess later. It also saves arguments between loved ones with differing views.

Joint accounts. Add the care partner or another trusted person to all of the PwLB's account—bank, credit card, even private savings accounts. Couples often do this as a matter of course. Both names are on their cars, bank accounts, etc. even though only one may drive or write checks. If the care partner has a personal account, add a trusted person to it as well. When someone must take over financial responsibilities, joint ownership makes the job much easier.

Lists. Make lists of everything that might be important later and show where these items are stored. Include IDs and passwords for anything online. Add any other necessary digital information such as a special word or phrase to use in case of a forgotten password. If a bill is automatically paid online or via a credit card, show that information. The lists should include:

Insurance and legal papers. Note when insurance payments are due, such as in January and July.

Pensions and other sources of income. Note when payments should arrive, how they are paid and whether they will continue after your death.

Real estate properties. Include physical locations, deeds, mortgages, insurances, and anything applicable.

Bank, savings, broker and other financial account. Include addresses, any automatic payments in or out and anything else that will help a person contact and use the accounts.

Credit cards. Card type, company, account number, the owner's name exactly as it is shown on each card and any other pertinent information such as expiration date, address, and online contact information.

Digital ID, passwords and any other information required to access online banking, social sites, social and personal websites or any other online sites that might need to be accessed later.

Fund Sources

A progressive debilitating disorder like LBD is always expensive. You may not need this information right away but it helps to be aware of it so that when you do need it, you know the various requirements. In addition to the following, the *Guide* offers some suggestions for financial support on pages 206-208.

Social Security. There are two programs, Social Security Disability Insurance (SSDI), for people who have worked five of the past ten years and Supplemental Security Income (SSI), for people who qualify for low-income status.[62] Apply at your local Social Security office. Be aware that you will almost always be rejected when the first time you apply, but will likely be accepted the second time. Consider getting help from a disability lawyer. There is a lot of paperwork and a lawyer can make sure it is done correctly.

Compassionate Allowance. Recently the federal government began a program that makes it easier for people with dementia to get Social Security Disability benefits. In the past, it could take up to two years to qualify. Now the PwLBD may qualify for benefits in less than two weeks. It requires:

- Documented evidence of progressive dementia from a doctor and
- Documented evidence of progressive loss of functionally from a care partner or family member, via an Activities of Daily Living (ADL) report.[63] Most insurances will provide their own forms but the Wikipedia[64] suggests a couple of forms to use if needed.

When documenting ADL's don't let pride or hope get in the way. Document your worst days, worst issues, worst problems, not your best. For instance, just one episode of not getting to the toilet on time and needing help to clean it up is enough to qualify as "incontinence." Likewise, one instance of "shaking so much he spilled food getting it to his mouth" is enough to say the PwLBD "requires help with eating."

Medicaid. Most states also offer Medicaid sponsored disability assistance programs and accept dementia as a disability. Usually, one must qualify for SSI and meet other state requirements as well. Medicaid is a low-income service. To qualify, a person must spend down their savings to only two or three thousand dollars. If a person or couple owns any property other than a home, this must also be sold and the money used up before they will qualify for service.

> *SSI Processing.* Expect to be rejected the first time you apply for SSI benefits. Accurate paperwork will go far in avoiding this.
>
> *Basic ADLs:* Activities such as bathing, dressing, eating, transferring, continence, toileting and mobility. Instrumental ADLs include telephone use, meal preparation, basic housekeeping and laundry, shopping, transportation, and managing medication, and finances.
>
> *Timing.* Get the long term care placement done prior going on Medicaid. If you wait, the choices will be fewer and the wait will be longer. Make sure the chosen facility accepts Medicaid, so that you can use it later.

Medicaid officials look back at finances for five years. This means that spending down funds by gifting others must be done at least five years before applying for Medicaid. For instance, if the PwLB has land he wants to deed to a family member, get it done now. Don't wait and be in need of financial assistance before the five years is up. Rules vary with states, and so check with a social worker to be sure.

The Federal Spousal Impoverishment Law. Also check to see if you qualify for exemptions provided by this law. It partially protects the income and resources of a person with a spouse in long term care (LTC). It allows a person to keep some income and resources. The amount varies each year and each state.[65]

Ask for information about these programs and any others in your community at your local Area Agency on Aging office.

Medicare. Most seniors use Medicare services already. It does not cover basic assisted living or nursing home costs like rent and meals. However, it covers a variety of medical and rehabilitation services, depending on the plan involved.

> *I found after the fact that Medicare would have paid for some of Bill's equipment, like his apnea hood. I didn't even think to ask at the time. – Marla*

Don't make the mistake Marla did. Be sure to check your plan before paying for treatments or equipment yourself. There will be enough expenses that won't be covered!

Veteran's Services.[66] If the PwLB is a veteran with at least one day of wartime service, he may be eligible for pensions, long term care assistance and admittance into a VA nursing home. See Veteran's Administration in the Resource section for sources with more information.

Warning: If LBD risk factors are already present, apply for long term care insurance BEFORE there is a dementia diagnosis—or if possible, even a MCI diagnosis. The price will skyrocket if you buy it later—if you aren't disqualified altogether.

Long term care insurance. This helps to pay for both home and residential care. Premiums increase with age and with certain conditions such as dementia at the time of enrollment.

At best, LTC insurance is expensive. However, it will save you thousands of dollars every month when it comes time to use it.

When choosing a long-term care insurance, consider the following:

What is the reputation of the company? After all, you want it to stay around and still be there when the insurance is needed.

What is the number of Activities of Daily Living (ADLs) where help is required before the insurance becomes active? The fewer of these tasks required, the easier it will be to qualify. Aim for only two and no more than three.

How long will the insurance pay for services? Many only pay for three years. Some are unlimited. Three years is usually enough, but if it is affordable, consider increasing time just in case.

Is there a built-in cost of living benefit increase? This will make the insurance more current with actual costs when it is finally needed.

Does it also cover home care? This may help the PwLBD stay at home longer.

What is the deductible? Most LTC insurance policies require the patient to pay for the first one to three months of service. Starting out with only a few hours of home care a day or week will make the deduction cost much lower than starting out in an assisted living facility.

Defining Dependence

To get certain assistance, meet the criteria for long term care, or for other legal needs, the PwLBD must be "dependent" and no longer be able to provide all of their own care. Geri Hall, the facilitator of a LBD caregiver's support group in Phoenix, Arizona, gives the following examples of dependence.

A person who is "dependent" may:

- Need reminders to do everyday tasks.
- Need things done for him that he used to do for himself such as cutting up food for safe eating.
- Need constant supervision and direction.
- Have episodes of wandering.
- Be a risk for falls or may have fallen.
- Have episodes of urinary incontinence.
- Have episodes of bowel incontinence.

Each agency will have its own requirements for which and how many of these conditions a person must meet to qualify. A doctor's evaluation of his condition may also be required. Due to Showtime, PwLBD tend to appear at their best in the doctor's office. To provide a more accurate picture:

Keep a journal and record all dependent or acting-out behavior with date, time and duration.

Talk about the worst day, not the best day, nor even most of the time. Often just one episode is enough to qualify for a particular condition.

Keep a careful record of all medications, administration times and positive and/or negative results. The doctor will want to compare medication and behavior.

Consider making video and/or audio recordings of confused, dependent or acting-out behaviors for objective proof.

Section Three:

Stress

Stress is not necessarily bad. It keeps life interesting and fulfilling. It is only dangerous when it exerts more pressure than there are resources to deal with it. Excessive stress increases the likelihood of many illnesses, including LBD. It does not cause these illnesses, but it can make it more difficult for one's body to combat them. Once an illness is present, excessive stress tends to make symptoms worse.[67]

LBD attacks the autonomic the nervous system (ANS) and lowers one's threshold for stress while adding the stress of living with a progressive disorder. Thus stress management is a priority. Below are three basic methods of stress reduction:

- *Control the environment:* Find the triggers and change the situation. Start by looking for the message in the behavior.
- *Control the body's responses:* Use the brain's powers to send calming messages, using a combination of knowledge and practice.
- *Build up the body's reserves.* Cultivate a healthy lifestyle that builds and maintains healthy brain cells. This raises the body's threshold for stress and increases the amount of tension a person can handle. Aspects of a healthy lifestyle are addressed in Section Five.

Chapter 18

The Stress Process

When a person perceives a threat, he processes it as an attack. He gears up to fight or run, whichever seems best at the time. However, many modern "threats" are not physical but emotional, where running or fighting doesn't work. This leaves the physical power generated for dealing with the perceived attack with nowhere to go. It circles back into the body and internalizes, putting pressure on internal organs and decreasing one's ability to handle stress even more.

Normal Stress

A healthy body responds to a threat or challenge by directing the autonomic nervous system (ANS) to increase the functioning of those parts of the body required for a "fight or flight" response. To provide the additional resources needed for the increases, the ANS sends more oxygenated blood to the organs involved.[68] These include:

The brain's perceptual centers. With increased awareness, one is better able to sense what's happening and respond quickly.

The circulatory and respiratory systems. Heart rate, blood pressure and breathing increase, so that more blood and oxygen can go to areas that need them for fight or flight. When there is little need, the increase appears as anxiety. In today's society where muscle strength is seldom needed, anxiety and stress are often synonymous.

The large muscles. Blood flows to the large muscles of the body so that a person can hit harder, lift higher, or run faster. When the muscles aren't used, this shows up as tension headaches, muscle cramps, lower back pain and similar symptoms.

To provide all that extra power, the ANS decreases blood and oxygen to areas of the body that are less involved with fighting and fleeing, including:

The thinking centers of the brain. Taking time to think while being attacked by a saber-toothed tiger could get early man killed. He needed to rely on learned responses. The modern body is still not designed for thinking to be a crisis activity. With less oxygen, the brain gets fuzzy and slow, making tasks such as creative thinking and seeing associations difficult.

The digestive system. Digestion is an ongoing process that can be sacrificed during times of crisis to provide extra energy for more needed functions. That's why a person may feel nauseous or constipated, or have diarrhea when frightened.

The immune system. Immunity is a long term process. It can be safely shut down for short periods, freeing up resources for more immediate battles. Shut down for long periods, it makes a person more susceptible to infections and other illnesses.

The threats that initiate a stress reaction can be internal, such as a broken bone or an infection. However, most of the time "stress" means perceived external threats. Fortunately, a person can make choices about how to process perceptions.

My boss told me that I had two days to complete the project. The worry that I wouldn't meet his deadline got me so agitated that I couldn't think clearly. And then I started

feeling nauseous. Maybe that's why it took me longer than it would have otherwise. I missed the deadline by a whole day.
— Lester

What is usually called "stress" is really stress overload. This occurs when perceptions create greater demands for performance than the body can provide. Lester perceived himself to be stuck with an unreasonable deadline. Therefore, he experienced increased anxiety and decreased thinking ability, classic signs of stress. His nausea was due to a disrupted GI system. His blood pressure was likely higher than normal too. His additional physical distress made meeting his already difficult deadline even harder.

My boss told me I had two days to finish my project. I told my boss that of course, I'd do my best to finish in the two days but that I believed that doing it well might take longer. My boss wasn't happy, but told me to finish as soon as I could. The funny thing was that I actually finished before the deadline.
— Beverly

Beverly chose not to be stressed and took steps to avoid it. Her functionality remained at a high level and she was able to finish her project on time.

Perceptions have a large part in what one considers stressful or not. Everyone chooses how to perceive life's events. Those choices affect your ability to make changes. You can choose to be passive and anxiety-ridden as Lester was, or like Beverly, be proactive which decreases anxiety.

Long-Term Stress

When the perception of threat remains and the demands continue over time, stress becomes even more internalized. This long term stress greatly increases the risk for most illnesses—infections, dementia, heart problems, diabetes, cancer, etc. Stress does not *cause* these illnesses, but it does prevent the body from using all of its own resources to deal with them when they appear.[69]

The more intense the tension and/or the longer it lasts, the greater the risk. As dementia or other illnesses appear, they tend to mask the initial stressor. However, if you can find and remove or change what was causing the stress initially, symptoms of the illness may decrease. For instance, decreasing stress can sometimes greatly improve cognitive function.

Lewy Bodies and Stress

Lewy bodies put a person at a high risk for stress and its damaging results. Early in the Lewy body journey, often well before any dementia symptoms are present, Lewy bodies begin attacking the ANS, making the organs it controls sluggish and less efficient. This lowers the stress threshold so that it may take only a little more pressure to cause an overload—only a small amount of worry, anger, frustration, confusion or pain. Lewy bodies build pressure in the following ways:

- What was easy becomes hard work, if not impossible.
- Perceptions increase, while the ability to sort them out decreases, causing illusions and delusions.
- Hallucinations and Active Dreams can occur, often with accompanying behavioral issues.

- Interpretation of feelings becomes distorted and impulse control decreases.
- Focus narrows; more than one or two of anything becomes confusing and overwhelming.
- Change becomes a frightening series of new experiences.
- Urinary infections, constipation, painful falls and other discomforts are common.
- Communication may become difficult or garbled.

With limited reserves, PwLBD soon reach the stage where they have more pressure than they can handle. The stress becomes internalized and symptoms increase, often along with anxiety, acting-out behaviors and infections. This is in addition to the same stress-related issues that anyone has.

All of this makes it imperative that everyone—the PwLB, care partner, family and medical community, everyone—work to maintain a healthy, low stress lifestyle. Starting this process early can make a huge difference in the severity of the symptoms.

Chapter 19

Changing the Environment

If you can identify what is causing the stress (the trigger), you may be able to change the situation to something more comfortable.

Identifying the Triggers

Likes and dislikes vary and so do stressors. Anything perceived as bothersome, annoying, threatening, or disrupting will add stress and when continued, eventually become too much for the ANS to handle. The same is true for PwLBD, except that with a much lower threshold, "too much" comes quickly.

If the PwLB already has MCI, now is the time to think about what is stressing and what is relaxing. As a team, think about activities, music, colors, and the like. Identify which ones cause tension and which ones are calming. Even at this early stage anything you can do to reduce stress will be helpful. Limiting stress tends to decrease symptom intensity and extend the length of time before severe symptoms become the norm.

Developing Stress Awareness

Stress is individual. What bothers one person might not bother someone else at all, and vice versa. While everyone reacts differently, the body's initial physical responses to stress are the same. Start by asking these questions about you and the PwLB:

- Is my/his heart rate up?
- Am I/Is he anxious?

- Are my/his muscles tense?
- Am I/Is he irritable?

These questions are not helpful for long-term issues, where the body has adjusted and internalized the stress in some other way, but your answers will tell you if there is anything immediate going on.

Stress is contagious. If one member of the team is stressed, both will be, thus the above questions are directed toward both members of the team. All efforts at stress management must be for the whole team. Your loved one will mirror your stress. He will telegraph his tension with behaviors that make your life more stressful.

Look for the triggers. Become a sleuth and look for what is causing the stress. This can take time and effort, especially if you tend to discount feelings or if the stress is long-term and therefore, less easy to identify. It can also take longer when you are the care partner hunting down your partner's triggers.

Each person's stressor will be different. It can be anything—a certain word or sound or sight, anything. Bill's was a word:

> *I always kissed my husband and told him goodbye when I left his nursing home at night. But he'd wake up in a couple of hours restless and agitated. I learned that if I waited until he was asleep and sneaked out, he might still wake up but he wasn't agitated. –Barbara*

Once Barbara figured out that the trigger for Bill's agitation was telling him goodbye, she understood that it was his body's way of communicating the fear that she wouldn't return. She changed her behavior and his stress-related actions stopped.

Look for:

- Fears like Bill's and their triggering words, phrases or events.
- Pain from infections, aches, illnesses or sores.
- Irritants such as an uncomfortable sitting position, wet clothes, hunger, frustration.
- Sensitivities to bright lights, loud sounds, touch or Lewy-sensitive drugs.
- Excesses like crowds or too many choices.
- Hunger, tiredness or illness.

Decreasing the Triggers

Once you know the triggers, you can make changes to remove or decrease them. Here are some common problems and suggestions for fixes.

Too many people. Due to LBD's limited focusing ability, the movement and commotion of crowds can become a jarring jumble.

> ***Fix:*** Avoid crowds. Learn when malls are least crowded and go shopping then.

> ***A more creative fix:*** Find a way to isolate yourself from the stressful hubbub of noisy active groups while still participating.

Ever since I was a kid, I've loved to go to the zoo. It's really crowded on a Saturday but Nick and I decided to go anyway. Nick brought along my ear-buds and MP3 player, so I could "tune out" kids and noise with music when I needed to. We stopped to rest in quieter spots so I could regroup. After about 2 hours I was beat; losing focus and balance...that happens when I get tired...but the ear buds and quieter places worked. I had a great time.[70] – Donna

Donna's MP3 player allowed her to spend an afternoon doing something she loved, even in a crowded atmosphere. Adaptation is the name of the game!

Sensitivities: Many caregivers report that their loved ones perceive light as much brighter than it actually is. Likewise, noise may appear not only louder but distorted as well, adding fear.

> *Fix:* Avoid bright lights and loud noises.

> *A more creative fix:* Use sunshades and sunglasses outdoors and even indoors if the light feels too intense.

Media, especially the TV: As the ability to differentiate between fact and fiction decreases, the PwLBD can perceive an exciting or scary television show as real and thus find it very stressful.

> *Fix:* Monitor the TV and make an effort to choose shows less likely to cause stress. Choose shows without a plot— sports, game or travel shows.

> *A more creative fix:* The Lewy team works together to select some low-stress DVDs to choose from instead of TV programs. This helps to maintain a sense of control while limiting opportunities for stress.

Physical discomfort in the form of illnesses, infections, injuries, constipation, and other irritants can be present and yet not always recognized as such. The PwLBD just knows he is uncomfortable and reacts accordingly. Find the discomforting trigger, fix it and the stress level will decrease.

Fears and other negative reactions. A damaged ability to communicate and impaired thinking skills work together to trigger stress. These problems arc addressed in other chapters.

Evaluating Your Success

Once you've found a trigger and made an attempt to change the situation, take time to evaluate. This way you will have a better idea of how to prevent or decrease that particular stress in the future.

In your journal, keep a record of your efforts. Answer questions like these:

- How did you know there was stress? Was there a certain behavior or action? What was the behavior's hidden message?
- What was the stressor? How would you recognize it next time? What can you do to keep it from appearing again? What did you do to change the situation? How effective were your efforts? What would you do differently next time?

Chapter 20

Preserving Familiarity

When your loved one's life moves towards dementia and starts changing in often scary ways, avoiding outward change and maintaining the familiar becomes critical. Once, variety and change may have been fun, exciting and enlightening. Now they move him away from the known, away from where there is still a sense of control. As the ability to adapt and learn diminishes, so does any appreciation of change. It is the enemy, stealing away feelings of comfort and security. Change and variety become stressors, while keeping everything as much the same as possible decreases stress.

As with other symptoms, this need for sameness may start well before any cognitive issues become noticeable. A person who has loved to travel may resist taking a trip, especially if it is to a strange place. Someone who may have loved to go to the theater may prefer to see a video at home. The milling crowds that used to add to the theater experience now cause agitation and anxiety.

Even if variety is still enjoyable, start now to prepare for when it won't be. Now is the time do some of the things that will be less enjoyable later—take that trip you've been talking about for years or buy season tickets to the theater. It is also the time to set up routines and rituals that will provide the PwLB familiarity later when change is stressful. And finally, it is the time to look ahead and see what else you can do to ensure less change in the future.

Familiarity can be expressed by actions and in one's relationship to surrounding places and objects.

Familiar actions. Routines and rituals are comfortable for everyone. Most churches use rituals to help members feel at home no matter where they worship. Mothers use bedtime routines to help prevent resistance. A familiar set of actions carries a person along to an expected destination with little effort. Doing something the same way every time may be boring for the person who thrives on change but not after dementia appears. Then, rituals and set routines have a soothing, almost mesmerizing quality that decreases stress and fosters comfort.

Developing routines for bedtime, eating, traveling and the like build in the comfort and safety of familiarity. If the PwLBD knows exactly what is going to happen, it is easier to take that next step—and the next and the next. Routines for activities like eating out will greatly increase his ability to do so with enjoyment. Encourage the PwLB to develop enjoyable rituals while that is still possible.

Familiar places. Home is the most familiar place and feels the safest and the most comfortable for most of us, and certainly for a person with dementia. Expand that sense of comfort by building routines of outings with the PwLB such as visits to favorite restaurants and stores. Take the same route in the car, ask for the same table at the restaurant, go through the aisles in the same sequence, etc. Building such routines now will make it easier to do these things later.

Places can also mean the location of furniture and other objects. Find the best placement plan now and stick with it. Every time furniture is moved, the PwLBD may become stressed—his sense of knowing just where everything belongs has been damaged and he feels less in control.

Familiar objects. Make less familiar places seem more inviting for the PwLBD by adding personal furniture, photos and other well-loved items. This works well when a move to assisted living is necessary. It helps at other times as well. Bring a favorite blanket or other item when traveling. The touch of sameness that it provides may make the difference between comfort and anxiety.

Buy the same clothes. If the PwLBD needs new underwear or a new jacket, buy something similar to what they've been wearing. Don't even change the color. The comfort of familiarity is much more important than style—or even functionality, in most cases. When you do have to make changes, don't make any more than necessary. For instance, Velcro-fastened shoes can help with independence. Go ahead and buy them instead of the PwLBD's old lace-up shoes but try not to change color or style.

Chapter 21

Changing the Body's Responses

The brain is a wonderful organ that can calm with soothing messages almost as easily as it excites with danger messages. The "almost" is because it does take a little more effort at first. Sending these calming messages isn't as instinctual as the flight or fight reaction that leads to stress. However, with practice it can become second nature. While the following suggestions are directed towards the issues that PwLBD have, these suggestions can also help the care partner choose calmness over stress.

Use compassion. This is usually easier with others than it is with oneself. When the PwLBD feels overwhelmed, encourage him to ease back on his standards, slow down, and treat himself gently.

> *A friend asked me to review her writing. I was glad to oblige. I've done a lot of proofreading in the past and I've always enjoyed doing it. But not this time. When there was more than a single comma in a sentence, I'd find myself going back and re-reading it over and over. I couldn't seem to get past those commas! I called my friend and told her she'd have to find someone else. This was just too stressful for me. — Jan*

Jan is just beginning to notice some symptoms of MCI-LB. Commas separate thoughts or ideas. Several in a single sentence triggered her cognitive impairments and interfered with her reading. Jan knows the importance of managing stress and so she didn't punish herself by trying to continue to do something that had become too frustrating. She gave herself credit for trying and moved on.

This pertains to the care partner as well. If you begin to feel you've failed, be as generous with yourself as you would be with someone else.

Use positive thoughts. Negative messages increase anxiety and keep the brain sending out those danger signals. Rephrase to make the experience positive. For example, change "problem" to "challenge"—something to make life more interesting. Encourage the PwLBD to say "It won't hurt to try." Instead of thinking, *"I can't do that anymore."* Trying and not succeeding isn't failure; it just means it's time to adapt. When the PwLBD takes longer to do something than in the past, encourage him to say, "I have plenty of time" instead of berating himself for being slow. Saying the positive statement out loud increases its impact.

Remove negatives such as "no" "don't" "won't" and "can't" from your vocabulary and encourage the PwLBD to do the same. Like Jan, he may find some tasks that used to be easy are now frustrating. Encourage him to say something like "I'm taking care of myself by cutting out unnecessary frustrations" instead of thinking, *"I can't do that anymore."*

Listen to music. Soft, easy listening music is relaxing for most people. Our bodies will slow down or speed up to match the tempo of the music.[71] It is also a part of many stress management exercises. Be careful not to let it be distracting however.

Exercise. Besides including regular exercise in your schedule, add a little more when you feel uptight. Encourage the PwLBD to do the same. For example, if he starts acting stressed, a walk around the block may help. There is a strong connection between exercise of any kind and stress reduction. It increases your "feel-good" endorphins, improves your mood, distracts you and becomes "meditation in motion."

Do deep breathing. Upon feeling stressed, stop and take some deep breaths. Taking slow deep breaths increases oxygen, which slows a racing brain and helps you think more clearly. Deep breathing can be done anywhere, anytime. However, regular practice is also important. Be careful not to hyperventilate by exhaling more air than inhaled. This results in dizziness and adds to the problem instead of reducing it.

Stress Management Tools

These tools also send calming directives to the brain. However, they usually take more training. For best effectiveness, they should be a part of a weekly, if not daily, routine.

Whole books are written about stress management tools. Colleges and community centers offer classes. Magazines and the internet have countless articles. Here are some suggestions to get you started. Choose one or two to learn more about. Then make them yours by using them regularly.

Muscle relaxation. Tensing and then relaxing muscles one set at a time from toes to head helps to consciously relax tense muscles. It releases the oxygen and energy held there and allows it to travel to places that need it more—like the brain. This is most easily done using an audio tape with guided muscle relaxations.

Self-guided relaxation: Think of a favorite restful place and put yourself there. One person may imagine they are sitting with their back against a shady tree near a babbling stream on a warm sunny day. Someone else might imagine they were lying on a beach near the ocean, or relaxing against a rock on top of a mountain with a gorgeous view. Combine this with some deep breathing for best effect. Guided recordings are also available for this type of relaxation.

Meditation: Sit in a comfortable position, close your eyes, breathe deeply and silently repeat a calming word or phrase like "Ommm" or "Let it go." This prevents distracting thoughts while you relax the mind.

Yoga: Perform a series of postures and controlled breathing exercises to promote a more flexible body and a calm mind. While often strenuous, yoga can be adapted to fit the needs of a person with limited physical abilities.

Tai Chi: Perform a series of slow graceful movements while practicing deep breathing. Tai chi is recommended for the elderly because the gentle movements are done standing instead of down on the floor.

With any of the above methods, also include the following:

Be consistent. These tools need to be used regularly. If one is not enjoyable, try another. This makes it more likely that you will practice enough to make it useful.

Practice, practice, practice. First response people like firemen or EMTs practice until their actions in a crisis are second nature. They don't have to think about it, they just do what they've learned to do. Athletes do the same. They don't become proficient swimmers or ball players or dancers without hours and hours of practice. They too need to train their muscles to act automatically. Practice a chosen stress management method every day so that when a crisis comes, you will be prepared. Practice so that reacting with calming behaviors is second nature.

Additional Ideas

Ideas for ways to reduce stress are as numerous as there are people. Here are a few to get you started—and they don't take practice. You just have to enjoy them.

Distractions can often tempt a brain to let go of anxious thoughts. Anything from eating, to a TV show, to taking a walk can be distracting. Be aware that if the stress is due to something physical, distractions are only a temporary fix.

> *Last week, Jerry's delusions got pretty bad. He was accusing me of all kinds of things. When it was time for dinner though, he came into the dining room and ate without a fuss. But as soon as dinner was over, he was back to ranting at me. That seemed odd and so I called Jerry's doctor. He thought it might be a UTI and arranged for me to take a urine sample into the lab. Sure enough, that's what it was. — Beth*

The distraction of dinner worked as long as Jerry was busy eating. However, when he finished, his attention went back to the pain that he was telegraphing with his behavior.

Hobbies, reading, or visiting with someone can refocus one's attention and calm down the brain. Like other more simple distractions, these only work temporarily when there is a physical reason for the stress.

Pets and their unconditional acceptance can reduce anxiety. The repetitive action of stroking a furry pet releases feel-good hormones that improve one's mood.

Section Four:

Communication

Communication becomes important as Lewy-impaired thinking and language skills add stress. Care partners must learn to recognize other modes of communication and less stressful ways of relating with their loved one.

People with Alzheimer's can usually talk well even late in their journey. They may not be as quick to respond because their thought processes have slowed down. They may repeat what they say because they don't remember saying it. However, their basic communication skills are still present. It is different for LBD.

Several early symptoms can result in communication difficulties. Upon retrospect, many care partners will say that these issues with communication were the first ones noticed. The problems can show up before cognitive impairment or behavior problems.

Communication is often thought of as being verbal. As LBD advances, other methods become important. PwLBD will use these methods and care partners need to learn to use them too.

Chapter 22

Communication Altering Symptoms

The symptoms that affect communication are seldom obvious at first. They show up slowly, insidiously moving in and gradually changing the way a Lewy team communicates. Initial problems may occur during times of stress. Thus, when the PwLBD most needs to communicate well will be when it is hardest to do so.

Language difficulties may make verbal communication so frustrating and weak facial muscles may make it so exhausting that talking isn't worth the effort. The symptoms are not always obvious. Slowing thought processes, growing attention deficits and apathy may be seen as boredom. Light sensitivities show up as sleepiness. Misinterpretations and inappropriate responses due to failed thinking filters become identified as character defects.

Language Difficulties

Word recall difficulty. While everyone has this "it's on the tip of my tongue" experience at times, it can be a regular visitor for the PwLBD and may be an early symptom. A person often feels they know the first letter of the word or even how many syllables it has, but the word just isn't there.

> *We loved to go on picnics as a family. My dad and I still do, although we usually just stay home and eat in the backyard. Recently Dad suggested, "Let's go on a, uh…Let's take our food outside and eat on that table out there." "Oh," I said.*

"You want to go on a back yard picnic?" Dad responded, "Yeah, let's sit at the picnic table." — Deborah

Deborah's dad knew he didn't have the right word and was able to talk around it to get his message across. Once he heard the word, he could use it with understanding.

Word substitution. Sometimes people use the wrong word and don't even realize it.

We used to laugh when Quentin said green when he meant blue or things like that. Sometimes it wasn't so funny. He once asked me for a chair and was mad when I brought him one. He'd wanted a step-stool. That was even before we knew he had MCI. — Beth

Quentin didn't recognize he'd used the wrong word. Usually, the substituted word or phrase will be similar in some way to the intended word. It might:

- Have a similar meaning: chair vs. step-stool.
- Be in the same group: green vs. blue.
- Start with the same letter, or sound: computer vs. counter.
- Rhyme: washing fishes vs. washing dishes.

There may be no apparent connection at all. The further into the LB journey a person is—or the more stressed—the more garbled the words are likely to be.

Other LBD-Related Problems

Some of the problems with communication aren't directly related to language.

Weakened facial muscles. Even when Parkinson's is not involved, the muscles around the face and throat may weaken. Muscles that control the voice may be the first to be affected.

> *Quentin's voice got so soft I could hardly hear him but when I asked him to speak up he'd tell me he was already shouting.* — *Beth*

Quentin was making the effort to speak loudly; it just wasn't coming out that way.

Thinking errors. LBD causes a variety of thinking errors. Some result in delusions as described in Chapter 12. Others are less obvious.

> *I had to be careful how I told Quentin to do something. He'd go when I said, "Don't go..." or sit when I said, "Don't sit." I guess he didn't hear the negatives.* — *Beth*

The subconscious brain, even when healthy, tends to ignore the altering prefixes to a directive—hypnotists learn that "sit" and "don't sit" often generate the same sitting response. It is the thinking part of the brain that recognizes these and uses them to better identify what is meant. Quentin's weakened ability to discriminate caused him to ignore the negative parts of Beth's directives and do the opposite of what she wanted him to do.

Slow thought processing. As the disorder advances, thinking gets bogged down more and more. The PwLBD processes everything very slowly—for others, that is. For them, their mind is racing a mile a minute trying to wade through everything that's going on. It's like a car stuck in the mud with the motor racing but hardly moving.

One evening, before we knew there was anything wrong with Bill, we took my dad out to dinner. I asked Bill if I could have his butter if he didn't want it. He ignored me, and just sat there looking at his plate. I'm easygoing and so I didn't push; I just went on eating and visiting with my dad. Five minutes later, Bill picked up his butter and put it on my plate. Years later, after his diagnosis, I remembered that and understood that he'd been processing my question that whole time. — Marla

Marla asked a compound question; one with more than a single idea to be processed: a) Did he want it and b) Could she have it. Such questions take more time to process because each component must be considered individually. Also, Marla's conversation with her father may have been distracting, making processing the request even harder. It could have been worse. If Marla had repeated her request or asked if he heard her, Bill would likely have had to start over.

Attention deficit. A PwLBD gradually gets to where he cannot focus on more than one or two things at a time.

Joel gets agitated when someone tries to talk to him when there is loud music in the background. I am also beginning to notice that he hates it when there's more than one person with him in a conversation. And don't go talking about too many things at once. — Ronda

Joel's brain can handle only a limited amount of input at any one time. It works hard to process that. An excess of information just doesn't compute.

Visual perception. PwLBD my simply close their eyes and appear to be bored or asleep. As LBD develops, visual perception becomes damaged. Many caregivers report that their loved ones are sensitive to light as well as drugs. Other visual perceptual problems include poor contrasts, colors that are difficult to distinguish and motions that are difficult to process.[72]

Other Physical Issues

LBD is not necessarily the only thing causing communication problems. If you suspect that the PwLBD has any of these or some other similar problem, have them checked.

Poor hearing can decrease and/or distort the sound of voices, making people difficult to understand. Even a healthy person can become isolated by deafness.

Poor vision can hide and/or distort visual information. Add LBD's perceptual problems such as hallucinations, and partial blindness can be very distracting.

Depression and apathy may make the effort to communicate seem too much to deal with.

Pain, infections and other illnesses will take priority and remove focus away from communication, adding stress and increasing LBD symptoms.

Chapter 23

Communication Methods

People use a variety of ways to get messages across. The language difficulties discussed thus far mostly pertain to verbal communication. As the ability to communicate verbally decreases, other methods become more important.

> *A few weeks ago Kevin started yelling and trying to fight me. I almost called 911! He doesn't talk much any more but he has never been violent. I wondered if he was having delusions but he wasn't making accusations. It was more like he was trying to fight me off. I gently asked him what was the matter, and that just made him worse. Then I tried touch. He has a history of ulcers and so I gently touched his stomach and asked if it hurt. He winced and then nodded. After I gave him his ulcer medication, he actually fell asleep. — Sarah*

Kevin's angry behavior was a form of communication. Before resorting to calling 911, Sarah tried to understand what his behavior was implying. She thought it through and checked her conclusions by using words, and then touch when words didn't work.

Intensity, words, touch, tone of voice, body language and facial expressions all convey messages.

Words. LBD symptoms impair verbal skills more than any other type of communication. Words are symbols we use to express our feelings and thoughts. People hear words and use past knowledge to interpret what their meaning. They respond internally with a feeling or thought, interpret that feeling into words, and reply. When LBD damages a person's thinking abilities, the interpretation steps often get missed or garbled. Words become either misunderstood or unavailable. Then when muscle problems make talking harder to do and understand, many PwLBD choose to talk very little.

Intensity. This reflects the amount of tension involved. The mode of communication may change but the intensity of the message remains. It affects expressions, actions and voice tone. A low softly voiced "I love you" accompanied by a gentle touch and a loud "I love you" accompanied by a frown have totally different meanings. As a general rule, the louder, more energetic or negative an interaction, the more stress it suggests.

> *Because Kevin's behavior was so intense, I thought something very serious must be going on. — Sarah*

Sarah was partially right. Intensity can be a guide to severity, but only if the PwLB's thinking ability is intact enough to judge the severity of his discomfort. Without that ability, he either hurts or he doesn't. He is either scared or he isn't. He is either angry or he isn't.

> *My mom, Victoria, and I were eating lunch the other day when she became very agitated. I kept my cool and finally figured out that she wanted another spoon for her dessert. Her spoon had a spot on it. It doesn't seem to matter what the problem is. Mom gets just about as upset about something simple as she does about something really important. –Julie*

Victoria's LBD has progressed to where her the intensity of response to everything is on the same plane. Julie must use other clues, like hand signals or body language, to guess what her mother is trying to communicate. Even though a PwLBD may not be able to adjust his own response appropriately, his intensity may still mirror the care partner's. Thus, Julie's effort to maintain her cool was very important. If she hadn't her mother's behavior would likely have escalated.

Communicating via the Senses

We use touch, vision, and hearing to communicate. These senses convey messages to the brain via a different route than words do. This pathway is less likely to be damaged and so the message gets through intact. People in general tend to believe their senses first before they believe words. The communication is feeling to feeling; it requires little or no interpretation. A person senses (feels) something which is transmitted to the brain as a feeling. The brain responds with a like feeling.

The senses also convey intensity. A care partner's sharp tones or quick movements can be interpreted as threatening. A PwLBD's similar behavior can mean extreme discomfort, as it did in Kevin's case—or not, as in Victoria's.

Touch can work wonders when words fail. Think of a baby's responses. Gentle touches generate coos and cuddling. Rough handling generates crying and stiffening up--withdrawing. Babies don't think about how to act. They just do what comes naturally.

Sometimes George gets all wrought up about something and the only thing I can do is hold him tightly and talk gently until he calms down. – Janet

Janet's firm hugging imparts a feeling of safety to George and he can relax.

Hearing (tone of voice). Janet's gentle talking emphasizes that her holding is caring rather than harmful. It may also be somewhat hypnotic, which is also very calming. If Janet had yelled at George while she held him, his behavior would likely have escalated. The softer, more calming the tone, the more effective it will be.

Sight. Body language and facial expressions send messages too. Make sure they are congruent with your words. In fact, use these actions to support your words. Use hand signals, smiles and nods to help the PwLBD understand what you say.

Communicating with Behavior

When other forms of communication fail, the PwLBD may act out with behaviors that can be angry, combative or resistive.

> *Don had been difficult for some time. I thought it was due to the renovation going on in the bathroom. He refused to do anything I asked of him and became angry easily. He curled up at the bottom of the bed to sleep. When he got a red bump on his toe, I thought he'd hit it on the foot of the bed. But then the whole toe swelled up. I took him to the doctor who determined that it was gout. We put a plan of immediate action into place to relieve his discomfort. He felt much better by the next day and soon he was back to his usual sweet self.*
> *— Hilda*

While the behavior is not a symptom per se, it can be triggered by symptoms such as hallucinations or delusions or a variety of other problems. In Don's case, gout-caused discomfort triggered the behavior that was his body's way of communicating. With the pain clouding his already compromised thinking abilities, Don was unable to connect cause and effect. He didn't know that his sore toe was causing his pain. He simply knew he was miserable.

Behavior like Don's is often an effort to communicate stress of some sort. Figuring out what is causing the stress may be a process of elimination. First, Hilda suspected that it was from the renovations going on in the bathroom. Since change can be stressful, this was a valid guess. Eventually, she recognized that his red and swollen toe was the culprit.

When behavior is viewed as a form of communication rather than a symptom of the disorder, drugs are no longer the first response. First, care partners can look for the discomfort the behavior is trying to express. What is the trigger? Pain? Discomfort? Delusions? Hunger? Lack of sleep? Boredom? When something fits, find a way to solve the problem. Once the PwLBD feels heard, the behavior may decrease just as Don's did.

Chapter 24

Better Communication, Less Stress

As LBD advances, thought processing gets bogged down more and more. The s mind races as it tries to process what's going on.

The better your team's communication skills are, the less stress there will be—with equally less frustration, anxiety and acting-out. However, by the time communication becomes a major issue, the PwLBD probably will not be able to change. It will be up to the care partner to adapt.

Avoid distractions. Lewy's attention deficit makes it very difficult to focus on more than one thing at a time. Anything can take the focus away from the conversation: TV, a bird flashing by outside, children playing, and so on.

Be front and center. Position yourself so that you are in the center of the PwLB's focus before starting a conversation. Stand or sit directly in front of the PwLBD for best results.

Limit electronics. Leave radios, TVs and other electronic devices off unless these noisemakers are actively being used. The background sounds may provide company for you but they will make thought processing more difficult for the PwLB.

Talk slowly. It takes time for the PwLBD to process words. Talking too fast makes words seem jumbled. Pause a little between sentences. Talking slowly also decreases your stress level and a calmer person is much easier for the PwLBD to understand.

Talk clearly. Most people are able to make educated guesses about words that are unclear. Damaged thinking abilities make it harder for the PwLBD to assign meaning to an unclear word or phrase, based on the rest of the conversation.

Don't interrupt. Wait until the PwLBD is done with a thought before speaking. Don't finish sentences or try to provide the right word. Both add confusion and increase processing time. Only supply words if asked, or if conversation has obviously come to a stopping point.

Use a normal voice. Dementia doesn't cause deafness. Shouting distorts words and makes you more difficult to understand. It also makes you sound angry and can add to the PwLB's stress level.

Keep it simple. Avoid abstracts and complicated sentences or thoughts. LBD makes a person's thoughts more concrete. Complications of any kind are frustrating. On the other hand, remember you are talking to an adult, not a child.

Limit information and choices. Think about what it would be like if someone spouted out information about ten different things to you at once and then expected you to be able to discuss any or all of them intelligently. Few people could do that. For a PwLB, it gets that confusing much more quickly. Make "no more than one subject at a time" the guideline. Choices should be limited as well.

Use positive directives. Say "sit down" instead of "don't stand" or "stay standing" instead of "don't sit." This way, the message is clear and the PwLBD can more easily respond accordingly.

Use vision, touch and tone. Supplement your words with the senses. Make generous use of visual aids like hand signals, facial expressions and body language. Use touch to make a connection and hold attention. Use a soft and caring tone.

Make your body language congruent with your words. Be sure your tone of voice matches your words. Remember that when your words and body language disagree, most people will believe the body language. This is especially true when a listener has even mild dementia.

Watch the intensity. Keep your voice and movements soft and gentle. All too often, intensity implies danger for the person with a damaged thinking filter.

Listening with Care

As communication skills deteriorate, the care partner must develop an attitude of supportive listening. When this happens, the PwLBD will feel more heard and the unwanted behavior will decrease.

Practice patience. It can take 30 seconds or more for a PwLBD to process words and come up with an answer. Although this processing time may seem like forever to others, the PwLBD is so busy processing that it doesn't seem long at all for them. They won't be able to understand impatience.

Practice an attitude of normalcy and belief. As LBD advances and language skills decrease, continue to see the PwLBD as a person, not a patient. It is important to believe that even though talking may be difficult, *understanding is still there.* In support of this belief, researchers have long said that comprehension is among the last abilities to go.

Listen carefully. Limiting distractions is equally important for the care partner, especially as speech becomes less clear. Focus wholly on the PwLB. This is not a time for multi-tasking.

Ignore the mistakes. Do not point out inaccurate substitutions. This tends to embarrass or confuse which adds stress—and still poorer functioning. Usually, you can figure out the meaning and simply move on. The exception is if you can laugh together about it. Laughter will smooth out the feelings of censure.

Look for non-verbal cues. As verbal communication becomes more difficult, these become more important. Usually, these cues will also be more accurate than words as well. A pointed finger, a raised hand, fidgeting, looking in a certain direction, shrugging and facial expressions are all examples of non-verbal cues.

> *Luke doesn't talk much anymore so it's mostly a guessing game for me. But he does use hand signals, like thumbs up or down for "yes" and "no."* — *Kendall*

Look for intensity. Early in the process, the strength of a PwLB's reaction can provide a fairly accurate reflection of comfort level even when the behavior is inappropriate or irrational. More force denotes strong feelings such as frustration, pain, or fear. However, as the ability to make judgments decreases, he may become unable to judge the severity of discomfort. When that happens, he is likely to respond to everything with approximately the same force and intensity is no longer a good guide.

Use your familiarity. People who have been together for a long time will find that they often know what is wanted with very little communication. You likely know the food your partner prefers, his most comfortable chair and the way he prefers to sit, etc. Couples have been communicating thoughts with no more than a glance for years. Keep on doing it.

Encourage exercise. The "Loud" part of programs like Big and Loud[73] help to strengthen facial muscles by encouraging people to practice shouting in a fun atmosphere.

Make togetherness the goal, rather than being right or even always understanding. Touch, smile, laugh, and enjoy.

Section Five:

Building & Maintaining Reserves

The introduction to this book stated that no one had found a way to cure dementia; that all one could do so far was to slow the progress of its symptoms. While it would be wonderful if there was more, slowing the progress of symptoms and making them less severe is no small accomplishment.

Some drugs have been helpful, but all too often they can cause other problems as discussed in Chapter 9. This section and the next offer a variety of non-drug methods and therapies that can more safely decrease the severity of LB symptoms and slow their progress, extending one's period of awareness and greatly increasing one's quality of life. In addition, the time of severe dementia and illness prior to death may be shortened, although it may be more intense. Most Lewy teams say they prefer this to a long drawn-out time of helplessness.

Unlike drugs, which one takes and then waits for them to take effect, these methods and therapies take work on the part of the Lewy team. You have to do your homework. You will probably have to make lifestyle changes. You will have to persevere when you'd like to quit. However, if you do you will feel as though you, and not the disorder, are in charge.

Start by building a reservoir of healthy brains cells. The more healthy brains cells a person has, the longer the more severe symptoms of dementia can be avoided. A healthy lifestyle goes a long way towards building and maintaining these cells and keeping them functional. It also raises a person's threshold for stress.[74]

A nutritious diet, routine physical activity, regular challenges to the brain and the enjoyable company of others promote vigor, alertness and contentment while helping to build a reserve of healthy brain cells. Managing weight, getting adequate fluids and sleep and avoiding stress and dangerous drugs helps to keep those reserves.

Maintaining reserves also includes careful monitoring of the Lewy-sensitive drugs described in detail in Chapter 9. The inappropriate use of these drugs can undo much of the good gained from a healthy lifestyle and other reserve building and maintaining measures.

The information in this section is just an introduction. There are many other resources that focus specifically on each area. The LBDtools.com store is a good starting point for this search.

Chapter 25

A Healthy Diet

Living a healthy lifestyle tends to lengthen the time before the challenges of dementia start and makes them easier to deal with when they do show up. This starts with eating a healthy diet.

A Mediterranean diet is associated with slower cognitive decline and lower risk of developing dementia.[75] The antioxidants, vitamins, minerals and fiber in this diet work together to help protect against many other chronic diseases as well.

Foods in a Mediterranean diet include:

- Vegetables, fruits, beans, whole grains, nuts and a little wine.
- Proteins sources such as eggs, cheese, yogurt, fish and a little poultry, but very little red meat.
- Unsaturated fats such as extra virgin olive oil or canola oil instead of saturated fats like butter and bacon grease.

Choose foods that are:

Fresh or quick frozen. These retain their nutritional value best. Quick frozen can actually be better than fresh because the foods are processed at their most optimum time.

Unprocessed. Processed food will often include less healthy substances such as white flour or corn syrup. Labels should show no more than two items besides the food itself. For instance, clam chowder can have two ingredients besides the clams, milk, spices and vegetables.

Raw, steamed or grilled. These do not remove nutrients as does boiling, or add saturated fats as does frying. Baking can also work as long as the oils from the meat drain away from the food.

Properly prepared foods decrease the risk of metabolic syndrome, a cluster of risk factors for all chronic diseases: high blood pressure, high blood sugar, unhealthy cholesterol levels and abdominal fat.

A Relaxing Atmosphere

A pleasant, peaceful atmosphere without distraction or stress helps to digest the food better. This becomes more important as problems with swallowing and digesting appear.

Keep the focus on the food and the conversation. Soft relaxing music can help to set a calm atmosphere but loud, intrusive or busy music or a television running in the background is distracting. Avoid arguments and even mild disagreements.

Nutrition

A balanced Mediterranean diet supplies most of the nutrition a person needs. Except for a daily vitamin and mineral supplement, it is usually best to avoid other supplements. Instead, get the needed nutrients directly from foods. First, nutrients in food are generally more effective in combating dementia than the same nutrients in supplement form. Secondly, unlike prescription drugs or even OTC drugs, supplements are poorly regulated. There are no laws governing content. You can never be really sure the label is accurate. Finally, certain supplements can be dangerous.

Many vitamins and other supplements have been suggested to improve cognition, reduce stress and improve general health. The following have shown the most promise:

Vitamins A, E, and beta carotene: Helpful in many ways in food sources, these antioxidants have not yet been proven helpful in supplemental form. In addition, they are fat-soluble and may be dangerous in large amounts. Choose foods with these nutrients and avoid supplements.

> *Toxicity:* Most antioxidant supplements are fat-soluble and cannot be excreted in the urine. Taken in larger doses than the body can use, the excess is stored and can become toxic, causing liver damage or other problems.
>
> *Incompatibility.* Since drugs taken for other illnesses may conflict with some nutrients or supplements, be sure to discuss that possibility with the physician.

Vitamin B: Can be useful in combating stress. Supplements of these water-soluble nutrients are safe in normal doses.

Vitamin C: Useful in boosting the immune system and preventing infections. Supplements of these water-soluble nutrients are safe in normal doses.

Vitamin D: This fat-soluble vitamin has shown much promise for combating several conditions from heart problems to dementia although it is not readily available in a normal diet.

Supplements may be helpful but consult the doctor first and take only the prescribed amount.

Omega3 fatty acids: Useful in combating diseases that are dementia risk factors and maybe even dementia. Add foods rich in these nutrients to your diet and avoid supplements. (Coconut oil is an Omega3 fatty acid but it is also rich in saturated fat, so it should be used in moderation. The jury is still out on how helpful it actually is.)

Green tea: Found to be helpful. Drink green tea regularly and add other foods that include Quercetin, one of green tea's active ingredients. Avoid drinking this fluid late in the day, due to its caffeine content.

CoQ10: Possibly helpful but expensive and can conflict with prescribed drugs. Use only with a physician's guidance.

Although supplements are generally discouraged, the following may be helpful and are probably safe, especially if used with a Mediterranean diet.

- Vitamin B Complex, to combat stress.
- Vitamin C, to combat infections.
- Vitamin D, to combat dementia and promote good health.
- Two or three cups of green tea to combat dementia and provide hydration.

Lewy bodies may lower a person's sensitivity to many things. This can include supplements; thus a "normal" dose may be far too much. Consult the doctor before deciding on dose size.

Chapter 26

Physical Exercise

Exercise has been shown to be better than any available dementia medication or supplement for improving cognitive and physical function, increasing quality of life and decreasing caregiver burden.[76] It increases blood flow, thus increasing the oxygen that fuels the brain. Make regular exercise a part of the Lewy team's routine. Naturally, the type of exercise you choose will depend on preferences, abilities and what's available.

Aerobic exercise. Activities like walking, bicycling and swimming increase heart function. Chair exercises work for people who are wheelchair bound or have balance issues.

Weight and resistance training. Moderate levels, 2-3 times a week help to build muscle, and healthy brain cells as well. Combining aerobics and strength training is better than either activity alone.

Yoga, Tai Chi, or balance ball exercises. Improving balance and coordination decreases the risk of falls, already common with LB disorders. Tai Chi is especially good for the elderly because it is done standing—easier for someone with stiff muscles to do safely.

Household chores. Tasks like sweeping, vacuuming, gardening, doing dishes, making the bed, doing the laundry or taking out the garbage count as exercise too.

Aim for 30 minutes of exercise, three to five days a week. Anything that keeps a person moving helps. Start low and work up slowly. Be consistent—don't quit. Choosing enjoyable activities will make it easier to keep exercising.

As with the nutritional aspects of healthy living, there are many books and articles about using exercise to combat dementia. The importance of exercise can't be emphasized enough. Find something that works for both of you, together or separately, and commit to doing it regularly. Don't quit. If a type of exercise becomes too difficult, adapt, but don't quit.

> *EXERCISE* is considered by most doctors to be better than dementia medication, supplements or anything else for improving cognitive and physical function, increasing quality of life and decreasing caregiver burden.
>
> If you do nothing else, make sure you both get plenty of exercise.

Chapter 27

Exercising Your Brain

There is a large amount of research showing that people who exercise their brains consistently throughout their lives are at less risk for dementia. If dementia does appear, it tends to do so later in life. Even with dementia, mental exercises improve one's quality of life and the ability to interact with others.[77]

Mentally active people, even those with MCI, appear to have a slower rate of decline.[78] Researchers suggest that such people build up a "cognitive reserve" that helps to mask encroaching dementia. When that reserve is gone, the course of the disorder will accelerate. Being mentally active does not necessarily extend life; however it does appear to extend awareness while shortening the time of helplessness, when dementia is present and active.

For better mental stimulation, try any or all of the following. Although the suggestions themselves are appropriate for both partners, the comments pertain mostly to the PwLB's special needs.

Take lessons. Has the PwLB always wanted to play tennis or the piano? Give it a try but don't make it stressful. The goal is to enjoy the challenge, not be perfect.

Read a book. Read whatever is enjoyable. Although reading is often one of the first skills to go, stretch it out by using large print books. Those using an e-tablet can enlarge the print. As concentration skills decrease, the larger size print makes reading easier. A short attention span, and possibly a disappearing memory, can make lengthy books difficult even with large print. Choose books or magazine articles short enough to read at one sitting. Children's books have short stories in nice large print. Although the content is seldom right for adults, reading them to grandchildren might be a very enjoyable exercise. The LBDtools.com store has some easy-to-read adult books.

Listen to someone else read. When reading is no longer possible—or even before, listen while someone else reads, then discuss what's been read. This exercises the brain twice—once when listening and again with the discussion. There's also a pleasant social aspect in reading aloud.

> *For years I read to Larry while he drove. I've continued to read, doing it at home now instead of in the car. He sits with his eyes closed. Sometimes, I think he's asleep but when we talk later, it's clear that he was listening…well, most of the time. He falls asleep now and then. When he dozes off, I just quit reading for a while. If he's awake, he will open his eyes and look at me like, "Why'd you quit?" We laugh, and I start reading again. Otherwise, I just stop and let him sleep. – Doris*

With a PwLB's super sensitivity to other stimuli, listening with eyes closed helps to maintain focus. As the disorder progresses, Doris will probably notice that Larry falls asleep more often when she reads. This need for more sleep is normal.

Play solitary games: Do crossword puzzles, Sudoku, play solitaire or any of the many activities that take only one person. One skill may leave before another. For example, the PwLBD may be able to do Sudoku with numbers long after he's stopped being able to do crossword or other word puzzles, or vice versa.

Play games with another person. This provides a chance for togetherness and socialization and allows PwLBD to be able to play the games longer. Even games meant for one person, like a crossword puzzle, can be done with two people.

> *Dean could play gin rummy and chess in 2006 and beat me....When those games became too difficult we enjoyed crossword puzzles together, and Chinese Checkers with pegs. When he could no longer focus on the pegs or small print, we played thinking games like Trivial Pursuit. We tried to answer questions as a team.*[79] *— Judy Towne Jennings*

Although LBD eventually decreases cognitive skills even with the best of care, Dean and Judy didn't give up. They continued to find games both could enjoy. Start with a favorite. When it is no longer fun, either change the rules to make the game easier or find a different game.

Plant a garden. If getting down on the ground is difficult, use a raised garden plot. Have fun playing in the dirt, seeing a flower grow and bloom, smelling the fresh air, and experiencing the feel of working with the soil. This is another activity to do together or with others—a grandchild, for example. Working on a mutual project adds a special feeling of communication without saying a word.

Do anything creative. If you have a craft or creative skill like painting or music, keep on doing it. Even though skills may degenerate as LBD advances, the enjoyment from being creative does not. Focus more on enjoyment than on performance. Several people with early dementia have written books. Others have used their art to communicate feelings even after speaking became difficult.

Chapter 28

Being Social

Humans are essentially social beings. People use conversational skills to let others know wants, express emotions, empathy, humor and pleasure, to be helpful and much more. Being able to communicate adds to one's self-respect and to one's ability to accept and be accepted by others.

People need to interact socially to thrive. A person who lives alone and has little interaction with others is at a much higher risk for dementia than someone who is continually interacting with others. Social activities such as visiting with friends or relatives, playing bingo, and attending religious services have been found to be as effective at warding off dementia or slowing it down as doing crossword puzzles or playing solitaire.[80] It's more than that. The ability to connect with others adds much to a person's sense of well-being and general quality of life.

While socialization often includes speaking, it does not have to. One can connect with another person with a look, a touch, a gesture, or even by doing a task together. If speaking is difficult, go walking in a crowded place such as a mall and count how many people you have to smile at before one smiles back. Smiles are communication too!

These suggestions work for anyone, with or without a Lewy body disorder.

Exercise with others. Exercise is helpful in combating both dementia and stress. Add a social aspect by joining an exercise group. Physical therapy programs like Big and Loud[81] are great for the PwLB's movement, vocalization and cognition.

Refuse to be embarrassed. Care partners can laugh when they stumble or forget a word instead of being embarrassed. It will then be easier for the PwLBD to do the same. Others will follow suit and will usually be quite accepting and matter of fact.

Enjoy. Make an effort to enjoy the people around you. It makes conversing with them easier.

Keep the stress down. The lower your stress, the easier interactions with others will be.

Laugh and tell jokes. Humor lightens things up, decreases stress and makes conversations flow easier.

Finally, don't forget to share touch and affection. Even when talking is difficult, this remains.

Chapter 29

Putting It All Together

The body is a unified whole. Improving one aspect changes the whole body. Exercise works well for combating dementia—and decreases stress. Mental and social stimulation each help too. The three work best when combined. For instance, problem solving while talking and walking with a friend is better than just visiting or problem solving or walking. Golf, tennis, bowling, dancing, walking, skating and skiing are just some of the many sports that also involve thinking and socialization.

LBD will eventually lower abilities. That is no reason to quit an enjoyable activity. Instead, adapt. Encourage the PwLBD not to quit until he absolutely has to. The following will help him continue to play longer.

Have fun. Participating in something enjoyable increases one's self-esteem and sense of well-being. It keeps one coming back to do it again and again.

> *Coy had his first golf outing of the season today. It was the first morning in two weeks he didn't beg for "just 15 more minutes" in bed. He had a reason to get up! At the golf course, they paired him with a volunteer and headed out. I can't tell you how thrilled we are that he can still have this in his life. It is exercise, it is fresh air, it is a little socializing, and it reassures him that his life isn't over.*[82] *— Jeanne*

Coy was motivated to get up. He felt alive and wanted to be active. Having fun is good therapy! Find an activity the PwLBD enjoys as much as Coy enjoyed golf, and help him continue to do it. Find ways to make it keep on being fun.

Change the focus. Encourage the PwLBD to avoid comparing his abilities now to what they used to be, nor to what others can do. That is too discouraging. The focus must change from perfection to persistence. It's not how good his game is but that he continues to play and how that helps him to be healthy and happy.

> *I used to play golf—I loved it. Loved getting out and playing the game, competing with the guys and getting the exercise. I was good too. One year I even won our local tournament. I don't play anymore. I tried a couple times lately but my game is way off. I wouldn't want anyone else to have to put up with me and besides, it would be embarrassing. I can't even make par now. — Ed*

It's not unusual for experienced players like Ed to stop when they can no longer excel. If Ed can change his focus from winning to enjoying the game, he can still feel good about golfing.

Change the challenges. The challenges are still there—many more than before, in fact. They are simply different.

> *I used to be a risk-taker, an "adrenalin junkie," seeking out thrills to fulfill my need for excitement. Now my disorder provides all the challenges I need.[83] — Charles Schneider*

A challenge is something that calls for special effort. Meeting a challenge increases self-esteem and builds feelings of accomplishment. People usually challenge themselves to work toward being "better"--better than others, or better than their own previous efforts. However, that isn't the only way to judge success.

> *I once watched a diving contest between people who had never dived prior to practicing for the event. The highest score went to a tall, skinny 65-year-old man who belly-flopped from the high board. Coy is like that guy. He may not do it well, but he just keeps on trying. I so admire his courage. —* Jeanne

The man won because the judges were evaluating success by the effort and courage it took to overcome adversity more than form; or by the journey, rather than by the end result. This is how the PwLBD must view challenges. It took Coy a lot of effort to continue to play golf, but at the end of the day, he knew he had met his challenge and accomplished his goal.

Adapt. With LBD, adapting is the name of the game.

> *As [Dean's] disease continued to work on his agility and stamina, his tennis buddies and I adjusted his playing time. Finally, Dean had to give up playing because his balance was too precarious. Then, he became an enthusiastic fan. The group continued to include him in their socializing. Their support was of tremendous benefit to his self-esteem.*[84] *—Judy Towne Jennings*

When the standard rules make playing too difficult to be enjoyable, help the PwLBD to adapt. When that is too hard, adapt again. The time may come when he will have to stop playing. Even then, he doesn't have to give up. As Dean did, become a fan, a spectator. That can be a physically and mentally stimulating activity as well.

Choose the right companions. Choose people who are playing more for the enjoyment of the game than for the scores. The PwLBD needs friends willing to play at his optimum level, making the challenge neither too easy nor too hard.

Dean's tennis buddies worked with him. So did the volunteer who golfed with Coy. A bunch of regular players might be too focused on scores. However, one or two of Ed's friends might be willing to play with him "just for fun." Of course, Ed would likely have to tell his friends about his MCI, often a challenge of its own, but well worth the effort.

Search for accommodations. Whatever the activity, there is likely some disability support in the community.

> *The most tiring part for Coy was getting in and out of the cart. The volunteers have special permission to drive the carts right up to the ball, so the amount of walking was minimal, but nine holes certainly wiped him out. — Jeanne*

Jeanne and Coy found a golf course that provided volunteers and accommodation for his disabilities. Whatever the PwLB's hobby, ask around and find out what accommodations can be made so that he can continue doing an enjoyable activity.

Diversify and vary. The brain works a little harder when it is not following a set pattern. Vary activities from day to day. If the PwLBD plays golf with his buddies one day, play word games with him another day. As LBD advances, variety stops being challenging and becomes stressful. Even then, a person can still vary the order of known activities. For example, if the

PwLBD does aerobic workouts, help him to vary the order of the movements.

Dance. No matter what other activities the PwLBD does, consider dancing in some form, even if it is in a chair. It is a great way to exercise brain and body and adds a social aspect as well. Music increases your ability to move, adds energy and triggers a different area of the brain than thought does. Most PD groups offer dancing classes.

Keep the stress level down. Anytime these activities cause more stress than benefits, the advantages gained from the activity are lost. It may be time to adapt the rules—or change the focus.

Chapter 30

Weight Management

Weight management helps to maintain and protect healthy brain cells. LBD related apathy, impulsivity, decreased physical abilities and a fading ability to connect cause and effect can make this normally difficult job even more trying. Weight gain and loss are both issues, but loss will eventually become more important. Always talk with a doctor before embarking on any weight change program, and that the choices support the rest of the PwLB's treatment.

Promoting Weight Loss

Obesity is a risk for most chronic disorders, including dementia. It strains the heart and lungs, making it more difficult to get oxygen to the brain, decreasing cognition. It strains the joints, making exercise painful and less enjoyable. Less exercise means more the likelihood of LBD symptoms. Lugging extra weight is tiring and discouraging, adding stress, which may also increase symptoms.

Become motivated. Rephrase "dieting," to "healthy eating," which is more positive. Find a support group with similar needs and goals, such as Weight Watchers or TOPS. People in such groups lose weight more easily and keep it off longer than those who go it alone.

The Mediterranean diet. This style of eating supports weight loss when it is needed. Remember it includes a pleasant eating environment as well as healthy food choices. (See the Chapter 25, A Healthy Diet for more information about this.)

Promoting Weight Gain

As LBD progresses, eating may become more challenging and less enjoyable. Malnourishment often becomes a serious issue. It can make a person physically and mentally weak, and increase susceptibility to infections and illnesses. Work as a team to find food that is both nourishing and enjoyable.

> *Priority change.* Whatever the PwLBD can enjoy will become more important than what is healthy. While that remains an issue, simply getting food of some sort down is the primary goal at this stage.

Small meals several times a day. Recommended for general healthy consumption, eating several small meals take less energy and effort than consuming two or three larger ones.

Enhanced flavors. Add spices as tolerated or try adding fruit, beef or chicken flavoring. If sodium is an issue, be sure to check the sodium content of the additions.

Semi-liquid shakes. Combine a variety of foods such as pureed vegetables and fruits, small amounts of meat, and mild spices with water, juice or milk. These shakes are easier to swallow than either solid food or plain liquid.

Liquid nutritional supplements. Many older adults find milk difficult to swallow or hard to digest. Liquid supplements such as Ensure or Boost do not contain milk, often making them easier to swallow and digest. Their high nutritional content can be helpful when getting enough nourishment via food is difficult.[85] If the PwLBD doesn't like one, try another. Each brand tastes different and has several flavors.

Chapter 31

Sleep

For the PwLB, sleep is a conundrum. The healthy brain needs rest to function properly. A brain with Lewy bodies must work harder and so it needs even more rest. However, this may not be easy.

Falling asleep and staying asleep at night may be easier said than done. Sleep disturbances such as Active Dreams, sleep apnea or restless leg syndrome can interrupt sleep. Excessive daytime sleep causes sleep rhythms to change and decrease nighttime sleeping. Therefore, it isn't surprising that LBD families clamor for a safe sleeping pill.

Sadly, most common sleep medications are strong sedatives and therefore may not be safe for someone at risk for this disorder. There are some alternatives however:

Melatonin. Talk to the doctor about trying this natural hormone. It triggers wake and sleep cycles, is seldom Lewy-sensitive, and may work as a sleep aid. A possible side effect is depression—another common LBD symptom. However, since the results will be temporary, it might be worth a try. If it does cause depression, try using melatonin in combination with bright lights, below, to decrease such side effects.

In addition, try these non-drug suggestions:

Daytime activity. Stay active during the day, even if it is an effort. A person who sleeps or just sits around all day isn't going to sleep as well at night as one who keeps busy.

Short naps. Especially later in the journey, too much stimulation during the day can cause night-time wakefulness. Consider an early afternoon nap to limit stimulation.

A calm, dark, airy bedroom. Have good air exchange, and a minimal number of blinking lights from clocks, etc. The air exchange makes breathing easier. Blinking lights can trigger confusion, especially for anyone half asleep.

A set routine. As with everything else, routines help sleep come easier for the PwLB. Include a set bedtime and the same few low stress, enjoyable activities each evening.

Avoid evening excitement. Watch soothing TV shows and avoid anything boisterous or argumentative, or even just stimulating. Such shows can trigger Active Dreams or nightmares.

Bright lights. Have bright light exposure during the day. A bright-light box[86] early in the morning might help to adjust wake-sleep rhythms. During the rest of the day, be around as much natural daylight as possible. Sunlight and bright-light boxes can also help depression. *Warning:* Be prepared with sunglasses to protect the eyes.

Medication time change. Caregivers often report that dementia drugs such as Exelon or Aricept taken in the evenings increase the likelihood of Active Dreams, nightmares and general restlessness. Ask the doctor if the time can be moved to morning. Likewise, anxiety management medications such as Seroquel may work best in the evening, when the calming effects facilitate sleep.

As the disorder progresses, a person tends to sleep more. Towards the end, a PwLBD may spend more time asleep than awake. Do not be disturbed. This is normal. Their body needs much more rest to function. The main problem now may be trying to get sleep cycles adjusted so that awake time is during the day. The techniques for doing this remain the same as those previously mentioned.

Chapter 32

Fluids

Fluids are as essential to the body as good nutrition, perhaps more so. They are also crucial for good cognitive health.

My mom, Joan, lived alone for years. Then I learned that she had stopped playing her beloved bridge—she couldn't remember how to bid. I visited for a week and discovered that Mom was hallucinating too. Her doctor said she was dehydrated. After I made sure she was drinking plenty of fluids, Mom's neighbors commented on how much more alert she was. But it didn't last. I was back home less than a month when a neighbor called to say Mom was getting worse. I packed up and moved in with her. If I hadn't, she would probably have had to go into an assisted living situation. — Judy

Joan's dementia was nudged into existence by dehydration. With the return of adequate fluids, her brain began to function better. However, she wasn't able to see cause and effect well enough to maintain her hydration alone; some of the dementia was residual. Eventually, Joan was diagnosed with early LBD.

The circulatory system uses water to transport nutrients and oxygen. The liver needs water to flush out toxins. Inadequate fluids make these already LBD-compromised systems even more sluggish. Joan wasn't getting enough oxygen to her brain and her liver couldn't filter all the toxins out of her body.

A person needs from four to eight glasses of fluids a day, more if active, if it is hot or if they are at a high altitude. Any fluid counts but some fluids are less helpful. Caffeine is a diuretic and causes you to lose much of the fluid you drink. Colas have caffeine. Diet sodas have sweeteners that aren't healthy in excess. Regular sodas add calories without nutrition.

Make drinking plenty of water a habit. If you like, add a little lemon, or even lemon and honey. Use green tea, rich in dementia combating nutrients, for part of your fluid.

> *Simple test for adequate fluid intake:* Check the urine. It should be pale yellow. A darker shade may warn of inadequate fluids. If keeping it light enough is difficult, monitor water consumption just as you would medications. (Some medications will color the urine. Check with the doctor to see if that may be so for you.)

As LBD advances, water becomes an even bigger issue than nutrition. The very real danger of choking can make swallowing scary. (See Chapter 8.) When a person risks aspiration (getting a foreign substance into the lungs) with every sip, they tend to take fewer sips. Thickened fluids will likely become necessary. Thickening agents are available in most health care centers.

Fear of incontinence or toileting hassles may cause a PwLBD to drink less. The truth is that when the body doesn't have enough water to function properly, both incontinence and constipation are more likely.

Chapter 33

Smoking, Alcohol and Marijuana

It is widely known that neither alcohol nor cigarettes are healthy. However, many people use these substances to make their life more enjoyable. Must a person who is losing so much because of a Lewy body disorder give these up too?

Smoking

There is some research that shows cigarette smoking may be helpful in lowering the risk for Lewy body disorders.[87] However, smoking increases the risk for many other diseases. Even if problems such as cancer, heart problems, poor circulation and diabetes don't kill you first, they all increase the risk for eventual dementia. Therefore, smoking in any form and any amount is seriously discouraged.

Secondhand smoking. The fumes from cigarettes are inhaled by everyone nearby. Care partners and anyone else in close proximity needs to avoid smoking or do it outside, well away from the PwLB.

Cigars and chewing tobacco. If at all possible, avoid all tobacco products of any kind. They all contain nicotine and many other dangerous chemicals.

E-cigarettes.[88] These newer electronic cigarettes are advertized as a safer, lower nicotine, alternative to regular cigarettes. However, e-cigarettes contain many other substances such as volatile organic compounds and chemicals such as nickel and lead. Electronic cigarettes should not be considered safe for someone as prone to drug sensitivities as a person at risk for LBD tends to be.

Alcohol

Drinking depresses the nervous system, already damaged by LBD. Therefore, drinking in excess or even in moderation is discouraged. However, a single glass of wine might be allowed.

> *I have early stage LBD. I really enjoy a glass of wine with dinner. Is there any problem if that's all I have? Deborah, my daughter, is worried that it might make the LBD worse. – Matt*

Maybe not. An occasional glass of wine might even be good for Matt. In the last decade, many studies have positively associated moderate alcohol consumption, especially of red wine, with a reduced risk of dementia and better cognitive function.[89] Therefore, allowing Matt this treat might be just fine. But first, he and Deborah need to understand what happens during sleep when someone with LBD has a drink of alcohol, so that she can be alert for problems. Let's start with a few basic facts about sleep, alcohol and the normal, healthy body:

Normal sleep occurs in cycles of 75% deep sleep without dreams, and 25% lighter, rapid eye movement (REM) sleep, with dreams. Each cycle takes about 90 minutes. A person may have several dreams each night but no one dream lasts very long.

Brian, a man with no major health problems, has a couple of after-dinner drinks while he watches TV. He says it helps him get to sleep easier. Alcohol is a sedative and so it probably does. It also will cause him to sleep more deeply with fewer dreams—

for the first half of the night. Then he may not sleep so well for the rest of the night.

That's because the body is all about balance. Brian's drinks lower the functioning of his whole system—blood pressure, everything. To compensate, his body secretes chemicals that direct its organs to work harder. Two to four hours into the night, the effects of the alcohol will be gone but his body's chemicals will still be circulating, causing a rebound effect.

Brian will be more restless and may wake up. In an effort to restore the ratio of deep sleep to REM sleep, Brian's whole night's quota of dreams will now be crowded into the last half of the night, resulting in more restlessness, and even nightmares.[90] A moderate amount of wine (two drinks) can increase restlessness and wakefulness during the second half of the night for a healthy person like Brian.

Now, consider Matt, who has LBD. His disorder has already made his digestion sluggish and so the alcohol will have a greater effect. Matt may respond to his single drink with dinner as though it were much more—putting him in at least, the "moderate" category. It will also take Matt a longer time to metabolize the drink. Even though he has his drink with his dinner, instead of later with his TV as Brian did, it may still have a similar nighttime sedation/rebound effect.

The effect of a single drink of alcohol lasts only as long as the chemicals are in the body. Therefore, Matt can try a drink with dinner. Then Deborah can observe his sleep pattern and behavior carefully. Is there more restlessness during the last part of the night than during the first part? If Matt's sleep pattern seems all right, is he more confused after his drink? If there is more restlessness or confusion, is it serious enough to worry about? If not, an occasional single glass of wine is likely fine. Of course, LBD is a constantly changing disorder and so Deborah should continue to watch for increased wakefulness. If she sees evidence of a rebound effect, Matt might try a wine spritzer with dinner, or have his drink even earlier, with lunch.

> *Aaron likes a beer in the evening while he's watching TV. I think it makes his Active Dreams worse. Could that be? — Jeanette*

Aaron drinks his beer later than Matt drinks his wine, closer to his bedtime. It will be more likely to wake him up in a few hours. Then, there's alcohol's effect on Aaron's RBD. With all of his REM sleep crowded into the last half of his night, his Active Dreams will be longer and probably more disturbing. Remember, even healthy people sometimes have nightmares. Aaron, who has RBD, can expect the same or worse. Jeanette is probably right. Aaron's beer is increasing his Active Dreams and he shouldn't have beer in the evening.

Before giving up his beer altogether, Aaron could try some adjustments. Maybe he could tolerate a half-can instead of the whole can. If that still affects his dreams, he could try drinking his beer in the afternoon instead of the evening.

For an evening drink, consider herbal tea or even a cup of hot water. Hot milk or cocoa have been regarded as soothing night-time drinks but the milk may be difficult to digest. If incontinence is an issue, avoid any drinks close to bedtime.

Marijuana

My cousin used medical marijuana for pain when she had cancer. She said it worked better for her pain than anything else and that she felt less anxious with it too. Maybe we use it with Dad who has PDD? He doesn't have much pain but he does have a lot of anxiety. It's not an anticholinergic and so maybe it wouldn't a sensitivity reaction. And it might give him some enjoyment too. -- Marcie

Marijuana is now legal for medical use in many states and for recreational use in several. Like Marcie's cousin, many people have found it helpful for pain and recreational users have always liked its tranquilizing effect. This has led care partners like Marcie to wonder if it might be safer for a PwLBD than traditional anxiety and behavior management drugs.

The few research studies that have been done show that it appears to help very little with anxiety and behavior issues, or other dementia symptoms. [91] The reviewers did note that it didn't appear to be harmful. However, the tests were done mostly with Alzheimer's patients.

For a PwLBD, it may not be so safe. While it is true that it isn't an anticholinergic, its use can make schizophrenia worse and may also increase psychosis in general, [92] i.e., symptoms such as hallucinations, paranoia and delusions. Marijuana is long-acting drug--it can stay in the body for five days or more. Thus, if a person does have a bad reaction, it may last for a long time. For these reasons, Lewy teams should be wary of experimenting with marijuana, at least until there is more research into its effects with LBD.

Section Six:

Alternative Therapies

Alternative therapies offer many ways to provide comfort, reduce stress, relieve pain and improve the quality of life with less use of Lewy-sensitive drugs. They include many ways already discussed such as living a healthy lifestyle and stress management. They also include the modalities offered in this section. While some, such as physical therapy, are generally considered a part of traditional therapy, they often work better than drugs.

Several therapies incorporate the building and maintenance of brain cell reserves that help to delay or decrease the effect of LBD. With any degenerative disorder, the goal of therapy is to foster the maintenance of still-present abilities. Of course, improvement can sometimes happen too, as when physical therapy leads to better mobility.

While these therapies can ease the LBD journey and make it more fulfilling, they are not cures. Learn to judge a therapy's success by how much the PwLBD maintains his status quo, not by how much he improves.

Drug therapy is covered well in the *Guide* and therefore, is not addressed in this book except for what was covered in Chapter Nine and the small amount mentioned here. The advantage of drugs is that one can often see immediate results, while most alternative therapies take time and effort to work. The disadvantage of drugs, especially those used for behavior management, is the possibility of drug sensitivity.

As a general rule, we advocate for dementia drugs and against drugs for managing behavior. That said, mild, quick-acting drugs are often needed to deal with immediate issues. Once the concerning behavior is less pronounced, non-drug methods can be tried.

Another exception for using drugs for behavior management is in anticipation of a high-anxiety-causing event, such as a move into residential care. Anxiety is like pain. If you catch it early, it requires less to keep it in control than it does to bring it down. Therefore, a short regime of a mild, quick-acting drug may avert the need for more drugs later--and make the event much less stressful for all concerned.

In most cases, the use of alternative therapies is well worth the time and effort they take, especially for the PwLBD who has already been sensitive to even one drug, and therefore is more likely to be sensitive to others.

> *Alternative therapies: Safer and often equally effective alternatives to Lewy-sensitive drugs.* Given the severe and often hidden dangers that many drugs may cause for people with Lewy body disorders, alternative therapies are highly recommended. They tend to be effective with many aspects of treatment, including stress and anxiety management, and tend to be safer than most behavior management drugs.

Chapter 34

Physical, Occupational and Speech Therapy

Doctors often use these three types of therapy together. Most treatment centers have therapists available who can set up helpful routines. Even if the Lewy team does not want to embark on a long series of sessions, a few visits to each of these therapists can be very helpful.

In the past, Medicare has paid for such therapy *as long as there was evidence of improvement.* It did not take into consideration the progressively degenerative nature of disorders such as PD and LBD. As of 2012, a new ruling[93] changed that.

PwLBD can now get ongoing Medicare coverage without fear of being dropped for not improving—a great help. Notice that this ruling applies to other services as well.

> *Medicare change:* As of 2012, Medicare *cannot* deny coverage for "skilled nursing care, home health services or outpatient therapy because patients have reached a plateau and their conditions are not improving."

Physical Therapy

If the PwLB has Parkinson's, you likely already know the value of physical therapy. While its primary purpose is to improve movement, any kind of physical exercise helps to maintain cognitive abilities as well.

These professionals know how joints and muscles work together. In just a few sessions, a physical therapist should be able to help the Lewy team build a home exercise program for specific situations and needs.

Physical therapist and LBD spouse Judy Towne Jennings used a strong physical therapy approach in her book, *Living with Lewy Body Dementia*. Her many helpful suggestions and lists are an additional bonus. This is one of the highly recommended books in the LBDtools.com shop.

Occupational Therapy

The occupational therapist focuses on how a person does the whole task, looking for strengths and weaknesses. Using this knowledge, the occupational therapist helps the PwLB find ways to continue doing personal care activities such as bathing and dressing, and other life skills such as cooking and money management, or even a hobby.

Speech Therapy

Many PwLB develop very soft voices and weakened facial muscles, sometimes before cognitive symptoms appear. However, they may not be aware of the problem. Talking takes as much effort as it ever did and it feels normal, or even loud, to them. A speech therapist can offer exercises that will strengthen these muscles.

> *When John started seeing a speech therapist twice a week, he did much better within three weeks. It was less tiring for me too—I didn't have to ask him to repeat himself so much. And*

John feels more confident with his voice stronger and louder.
— Pat Snyder[94]

Better confidence is a common and valuable effect of better communication.

When I mentioned that John was choking when he ate, his therapist trained us both in proper swallowing techniques. She told John that swallowing issues could send him to the hospital and he needed to take this very seriously. As soon as we started to do as she said, John's choking sounds disappeared from our mealtimes. Wow! I was impressed to see that it worked so well--and so quickly. — Pat Snyder

Many PwLB also have problems with swallowing. This can be a life-threatening situation. Food aspirated into the lungs can cause pneumonia, one of the most common and most dangerous complications of LBD.

Chapter 35

Music Therapy

Researchers have found that music therapy works well with Alzheimer's patients[95] and that it can be even better than physical therapy in helping Parkinson's patients improve motor control.[96] There has been no specific research with LBD, but care partners repeatedly report that it works well with their loved ones.

Music wakes up memories and increases alertness, with the effects lasting long after the session is over. Listening to favorite songs increases the ability—and the inclination—to talk. Music fights depression, a common LBD symptom. However, like any other therapy, this isn't a one shot fix. To maintain any gains, therapy must continue.

One of the last areas of the Alzheimer's brain to atrophy, the prefrontal cortex houses a hub that links familiar music, memories and emotion. Thus, music evokes emotion and memories until very late in the dementia journey, even after other means do not succeed.[97]

Frontotemporal Dementia attacks the prefrontal cortex first. Music is less helpful for people with this disorder as they have fewer emotions to connect to the music.[98] PwLBD never completely lose the ability to feel emotions. Like PwAD, they benefit from music's connection between feelings and past experiences.

While a professional therapist is helpful, a lay person—a care partner, staff or even an early LBD patient—can provide music therapy with only a little effort and training. As with everything that helps with dementia, the earlier and the more music is included in one's daily life, the better it works. While it does not cure or stop dementia, it can improve awareness at the moment and increase one's quality of life.

Have songfests. Sing together or if necessary, alone—but sing!

Be consistent. Be as diligent about this exercise as you are about physical exercise and good nutrition.

Have patience. Don't expect improvements immediately. It may take several sessions to see changes.

Choose familiar tunes to make an individualized playlist. Play the PwLB's favorite melodies. Choose a variety, with some slow and some fast—but not so fast it causes agitation. The choices will differ with each person and may take a little trial and error before you get it right. Start with the most popular songs in the years when the PwLBD was between the ages of seven and nineteen. Add any songs you know the PwLB enjoys.

Use an iPod or mp3 player with the above playlist. Do not use radio or TV. This often becomes background noise that agitates more than it calms.

Make music a tool to facilitate the proper mood for an activity. Use soft, relaxing music to counter agitation. Use music with a good rhythm for movement.

Chapter 36

Professional Counseling

Any time a family goes through major life changes, professional counseling can be helpful. Receiving a diagnosis of PD or LBD generates stress, as does living with the disorder and the changes that keep coming. You find yourself dealing with issues you don't know much about and don't know how to handle. You grieve the loss of your life prior to the overshadowing cloud of the unwanted changes. You experience all the feelings involved with grief over and over and wonder if it will ever end. The disorder turns everything topsy-turvy and affects relationships as well.

> *Mostly we get along all right, even though a year with LBD has limited George's abilities. He's still "George" and we can still enjoy each other. Right now, our main problem is that he used to pay our bills. When he started making mistakes I had to take it over. Now, he's angry at me for taking his job away. I feel resentful that I have to do something I never wanted to do and then, I don't get any appreciation—worse, I get yelled at. — Janice*

George and Janice are ideal candidates for professional counseling.

Pat and John Snyder[99] saw a counselor. She reported that they learned how to how to communicate better so that each of was actually hearing and appreciating the other's words--and feelings. "Counseling has given me better clarity," John told her.

Here are a few guidelines:

Attend as a team. Dealing with a Lewy body disorder is a team affair. Both members need to learn how to communicate better with each other. Each team member may also need individual sessions to deal with more personal issues.

Start early. The sooner you start, the more your loved one can be an active participant in the counseling sessions.

Choose the right counselor. Find a professional who is used to working with the grief and adjustments related to debilitating disorders. You also want one who works well with couples. Both will be major issues.

Combine. Choose a counselor who will incorporate your experiences with support groups, spiritual and other supportive sources in the sessions.

Strength, not weakness.

Some people believe that sharing their emotional problems with a counselor is a sign of weakness. Not so. Any debilitating disorder brings with it a new way of living, new challenges and new adjustments. Just as physical therapy helps a team adjust to new physical challenges, psychological counseling helps the team adjust to new emotional challenges. A team stays strong by using all the support available to them.

Chapter 37

Spirituality

Spirituality is a way of life. It can also be a valuable form of therapy.[100] Spirituality expresses itself through a variety of positive feelings such as gratefulness, joy and awe that combat the depression so common with LBD families.

Like music, spirituality is personal. Unlike drugs, it is free and you don't have to worry about dangerous side effects. No one needs to show you how to do it, although ministers, rabbis, priests and the like can be helpful. Whatever the team's beliefs, incorporate spirituality into your care plan, not only for the PwLB but also for the care partner as well.

Include spiritual beliefs in counseling. If you are doing psychological therapy, ask the counselor to take your team's spiritual beliefs into consideration when making suggestions. You will resolve issues at a deeper level of understanding and make the resolutions longer lasting.

Make spirituality a stress management tool. You will feel less burdened and find it easier to relax. Trust in a higher power can lower worry and stress, making it easier to deal with the uncertainty that LBD brings.

Reach out to your team's spiritual community. Ask the leader for support. Besides regular services, there may be counseling, member visits to decrease isolation, transportation and many other services.

I knew we needed help but I didn't know where to go or who to ask. I went to our pastor and asked what I should do. She suggested that I talk to the women's group. I didn't want to accept charity, but she helped me see that accepting help was a gift as much as the giving of the help. The women really came through for us. Someone comes and sits with Evan at least once a week so I can go shopping, or even to the prayer meetings. I hadn't been able to get to church much so that is a real blessing. I am so grateful to these women. — Lois

Include spiritual beliefs in your daily life. Say grace at the table. Read a daily motivational selection. Meditate. Pray. Do whatever helps you to feel spiritually connected. Don't let spirituality fall by the wayside as you grapple with these new challenges.

Chapter 38

Aromatherapy

Aromatherapy is the use of smell to trigger various emotions. It has been shown to have positive effects on reduction of behavioral and psychological symptoms of dementia. It is also believed to improve cognitive functions, enhance one's quality of life and increase one's ability to perform activities of daily living.[101] All of this adds up to a reduction of stress.

The sense of smell is closely connected to emotions. Some scents can excite and others relax. It is also closely connected to memory. Like music, it can be a strong trigger of memories, and can evoke reminders of happy times in the past.

An advantage of aromatherapy is its convenience. It doesn't require a specialist and can be done at home with comparative ease. The scents come in essential oils. When airborne, via a cool mister, diffuser or other method, the aromas are inhaled. This causes receptors in the brain to be stimulated.[102]

Many scents help to relieve tension and stress. Lavender is most recommended but chamomile, sage and geranium also help. These scents can be blended together. They can be added to a diffuser or mixed with cocoanut oil for massage.

Many PwLB tend to lose their sense of smell early in their journey. Even so, aromatherapy may still be helpful. Therapists have found that the healing power of essential oils is absorbed through the sinuses and into the blood stream weather or not the person can smell.[103] In addition, researchers have found that there are olfactory (smell) receptors in many areas of the body, including the skin.[104] If a person cannot smell:

- Consider using essential oils with massage.
- Use the same amount of oil as if the person could smell. Do not increase the amount.

Here are some easy suggestions to get started using an essential oil:

- *Bathe in it.* Put 4-7 drops of essential oils in tub *after* you've run the water.
- *Use it as a compress.* Soak a hand towel or wash cloth in warm water with a few drops of a preferred essential oil and lay it on the back of the neck.
- *Inhale it.* In public, put a few drops on a cotton ball and inhale deeply.
- *Avoid candles.* Candles come in many lovely scents. However, open flames should not be used around anyone with even mild dementia.

Aroma therapy is:

Simple. It takes very little work to prepare and use.

Quick: Because breathing in the scents gets them to the brain very quickly, results will also be rapid.

Effective: Depending on the scent used, it can calm or energize.

Safe: If there is a reaction, simply stop the therapy and the reaction will end.

Useful even if the sense of smell is compromised.

Chapter 39

Pet Therapy

Dad's little dog stayed with him practically 24-7. During the day, Gizmo sat on Dad's lap in the easy chair in the living room, and at night, slept right beside him. When Dad had guests, he always had something to talk about. He could easily make conversation about the dog, while remembering current events or previous visits were more difficult for him. In addition to the love she provided, Gizmo also became Dad's smallest caregiver. On many occasions, she sounded the alert that help was needed. Once, when Dad was struggling to get out of the bed while Mom was making breakfast, Gizmo ran into the kitchen and barked until Mom went to see what was wrong. [105] — *Mary Pat*

Mary Pat's story is repeated in different forms by many PwLBD and their families. Although a true "therapy pet" has special training, any well-mannered pet can provide wonderful therapy. On the other hand, an animal that is nervous, snappy, or poorly trained can cause more problems than it solves. A dog's amenable, sociable natures make them the best candidates for therapy pets.

This type of therapy isn't for everyone. The PwLB needs to be willing to bond with the dog. Care partners need to enjoy dogs as well because taking care of a pet adds one more responsibility to an already full schedule. In addition, the home needs to be pet friendly and have adequate space for the animal to move around. For instance, most residential care facilities allow pets on a limited basis if at all.

Having a therapy dog for the PwLB or anyone with encroaching dementia is similar to having a service dog with one exception: the care partner must be involved. Right from the first, you must learn to be a facilitator for the other two. This will eventually mean taking care of many of the dog's physical needs. If training is available, it should start as early in the journey as possible so that learning is easier.

If training isn't available or possible, gentle, well-behaved dogs such as Gizmo often take very naturally to being "miniature caregivers" without formal training. Trained or simply good pets, these animals can provide hours of unconditional love. Here are some other benefits:

Less isolation. Dogs are social animals and people are attracted to them—and by proximity, to their owner.

Less stress and depression with increased clarity. The dog's unconditional acceptance tends to reduce anxiety and agitation, which decreases LBD symptoms, including confusion.

Increased companionship. There's always a friend nearby, reducing loneliness and making life more pleasant.

Increased activity and sense of value. Pet care, including walking, grooming, and playing with the animal as able make exercise fun. Being responsible for pet-related chores adds self-confidence and a sense of being needed.

Chapter 40

Touch Therapy

Several small studies have found that the ancient methods of acupuncture and acupressure decrease anxiety, agitation, and stress. [106],[107] They often work better than the more modern medical methods of our Western world with no drug-related side effects. Massage and gentle touch have been found helpful with dementia. The evidence from caregivers is also positive. In all cases, results occur only with regular use and cease soon after the treatments end.

Acupuncture: A form of alternative medicine that treats patients by insertion and manipulation of needles at strategic points on the body.

Acupressure: The application of pressure on the same strategic points on the body to control various symptoms.

Massage: The therapeutic practice of manipulating the muscles and limbs to ease tension and reduce pain.

Gentle touch: The use of touch for communication of caring and direction.

Acupuncture[108]

I still get around well and I'm self-sufficient although I sometimes have problems talking. Clara wanted me to try acupuncture. I wasn't very into it but I did it just to please her. We were both amazed. It really was easier to talk. I started out going every Wednesday. By Sunday, Clara was having trouble understanding me again. We increased the treatments to twice a week and that carried me over. I'd been having treatments for six months when our daughter had a baby. We left home and stayed with her for a month so Clara could help out. By the time we returned, my speech problems were back. When I quit going, it stops working. — Carlton

Similar stories, especially from caregivers abound, with reports that acupuncture:

- Relieves anxiety, agitation, tension and stress
- Improves sleep and speech
- Decreases anger, combativeness and acting-out

On the negative side:

- Treatment requires a trained and certified professional.
- Results are temporary. Treatment must be administered at least weekly and the results disappear if treatments stop.
- Treatment can be expensive and is not always covered by insurance.
- The treatment's intrusive nature might be frightening to a person who is unable to understand why someone is inserting needles into their skin, even though they don't hurt.
- The patient has to lie still for 20-30 minutes. This might be difficult for some to do.

Acupressure

This therapy[109] is very similar to acupuncture except that needles aren't used. Instead hand pressure stimulates the strategic points in the body. Used appropriately, acupressure appears to provide help similar to that of acupuncture for:

- Relieving anxiety, agitation, tension and stress
- Improving sleep
- Decreasing anger, combativeness and acting-out

Acupressure is mild and non-intrusive, which gives it some advantage over acupuncture for the average LBD family. It is:

- Easier to use and less frightening.
- Safe for non-professionals to use. Care partners can learn to do it at home and care staff can learn to provide it in residential facilities.
- Less expensive.

Disadvantages:

- The milder treatments wear off sooner. Maintaining results may require several sessions per week or even daily.
- Professionals do have more training and background knowledge and may be able to do a better job. However, acupressure is seldom covered by insurance.

Massage

Massage therapy[110] can treat the whole body or just certain areas. Light touch can sometimes be more effective than words. Care partners report that it works well for:

- Relaxation and sleep improvement.
- Anxiety, agitation, tension and stress reduction.
- Pain reduction. Massage is especially helpful if the pain is from tense muscles.

Advantages:

- Care partners can learn to do basic massage at home.
- Gentle massaging can be a time of togetherness between care partner and loved one.

Disadvantages:

- Results are temporary and require ongoing, sometimes daily, use.
- Deep muscle massage requires strength and stamina a care partner may not have.
- A professional masseuse has more training and strength but treatments may not be covered by insurance or may be covered only for a limited time.

Gentle Touch

Touch addresses a different communication route in the brain than words. It can:

- Convey feelings such as care, concern or love.
- Provide direction by gently pulling the attention back to the job at hand.

Disadvantages:

- Can be seen as threatening when uninvited.
- May be distracting when used at an inopportune time.
- Can be felt as an attack when the touch is not soft or gentle enough.

Summary: Although acupuncture may work better for stress reduction and related issues, its disadvantages may make it less attractive to the home-based care partner than acupressure or massage. With some basic training, either of these therapies may be useful for treating stress related issues that otherwise might require medication. If medication is still required, the dosage needed will likely be decreased.

> *Gentle touch* should be—and usually is--included in every care partner's repertoire and practiced daily.
>
> Other touch therapies can also add quality of life and should be considered seriously.

Section Seven:

Your Support System

Dealing with any progressive disorder is easier with a strong support system. Don't try to do this alone. Don't try to keep it a secret. Do reach out to others. You will be amazed at the response when you are straightforward and honest. People like to help but they don't always know what is needed. Don't act like a victim, but do let people know you need some support in this journey you and the PwLBD are traveling.

Don't keep it a secret. Some people are embarrassed to have a Lewy body disorder. It is no more worthy of embarrassment than heart disease or diabetes, simply less understood. Instead of being embarrassed, make an effort to spread awareness. Most people are quite interested in finding out more about this lesser known disorder.

One of the most stressful problems that a Lewy team faces is a family member or other important person in their lives who resists the whole idea of LBD. The disorder's unique fluctuations can make it easier for that person to maintain their resistance. It is important that you and your loved one talk with family members about what is happening, what to expect in the future and what you are doing to extend the time before LBD takes control. If you are open, they will likely be less resistant and more helpful.

Be a teacher. It has only been 19 years since Lewy body dementia was deemed a formal disease. An amazing number of people, including medical personnel, have still never heard of it. Others don't know that it is more closely related to PD than to Alzheimer's. Like it or not, care partners often find it necessary to teach. Your job is to let those around your team know what to expect and what kind of support you need. Teaching is part of doing everything you can to develop a strong support system.

Many PwLBD become teachers as well. Some people with early dementia have written books that help others understand a little better what it is like inside their head and body. Others teach by example. Bill and Barbara Hutchinson traveled the nation, talking about LBD. Barbara talked but Bill was there at every meeting, a living example of what LBD does to a person and how to handle it.

Reach out to others. Reaching out for support is a sign of strength, not weakness. Most people deem it smart to use doctors for medical help and physical therapist for help with physical adjustments. It is equally smart to utilize social support. Such support keeps the team functioning better and longer.

Find support groups, supportive friends and community organizations who offer support. Use all the assistance available. This is not an easy task you have before you and you can make it easier by finding people and groups who will share the load. There are many. You just have to be willing to reach out.

Chapter 41

Support Groups

A support group offers anyone dealing with something as life-changing as LBD a forum for learning and sharing with others who are on the same journey that you are. You can vent and they understand. You can laugh and make dark jokes and they will laugh with you. A good support group is one of the best stress relievers there is.

If the PwLB has Parkinson's you likely know about support groups and how valuable they are for maintaining a healthy life style. The programs the PD community offers such as "Big and Loud" are well worth your team's participation. This book's Resources Section includes Parkinson's disease organizations with contact information. There are a multitude of these organizations. If you don't already have a home group, find a PD organization that offers support groups in your community, then call for times and places. Your team doesn't have to limit itself to one organization. Check out several to see what services they offer and which groups you like best.

Some PwLB don't have Parkinson's. Still consider connecting with a PD organization and maybe even attending some PD support groups just to take advantage of the programs. The PwLB may not relate with these groups, which often have a heavy emphasis on physical activity and physical therapy. However, keeping physically active helps to maintain cognitive function just as much as it does mobility.

Eventually, you may want to help the PwLB find a support group especially for folks with early LBD. These are more difficult to find. He may have to settle for a virtual group. The LBDA offers a virtual group for people with dementia on their forums in their Find Support section. The Resource section in the back of this book offers a list of other online support groups for people with any kind of early dementia.

The care partner also has special needs and issues. A support group just for you is more a necessity than a luxury. Read more about this in Section Ten.

Chapter 42

Family and Friends

As dementia gets closer, family is going to become more important. Reach out to family members, especially those who live close by. Is there extended family around that you keep saying you are going to go visit but don't? Call and invite them over.

As cognitive issues increase, isolation becomes a major issue. Make an effort to help the PwLB expand his core group of friends while he still can. Eventually, close family members and these friends are going to be the only people with whom he feels comfortable or even safe. The larger this group is, the less isolation there will be.

Encourage friends and neighbors to visit. Invite them to come and play cards, to watch a movie, to dinner or to simply come and visit.

Randy has always enjoyed having friends come to visit but now that his MCI has become more noticeable, he is a little sensitive about it. We still invite friends over. Of course, they know about Randy's PD—it's been going on for years. Randy has been good about casually sharing that MCI is his latest PD symptom and that it's likely to get worse. "But," I always chime in, "One of the ways we are combating it is by being more sociable. Isn't it great that something this fun is actually treatment?" And then we all laugh. That's good treatment too! —Evelyn

If possible, it is best if the PwLB can share the information about his disorder, as Randy did. Being upfront will help him feel more in control. Evelyn's comment gives visitors a chance to feel as though they are being helpful, and the laughter lightens the whole conversation.

> *Decreasing Isolation:* To limit the isolation becomes a major issue as cognitive abilities decreases, start early in the journey. Enlist the help of friends and family to begin building routines that include them.

Develop Routines with Family and Friends

Routines add a sense of continuity to a PwLBD's life. They make it easier to know what to expect. They can also make it easier for a caregiver to add needed respite into the teams schedule.

As dementia creeps up, the PwLBD will become more dependent. This is natural, to be expected. Without respite, it can take a toll on the care partner. However, LBD makes it difficult for the PwLBD to recognize or understand that. When routines are already in place, the PwLBD will be able to accept them as a part of what is expected, and even look forward to them.

As you develop routines, include some outings with family and friends. While these routines will make these outings enjoyable longer, attention deficit can make focusing on more than a few people difficult. Resolve this by limiting the number of people involved to no more than three besides the PwLB. The same problem makes listening to more than one person at a time difficult. Resolve this by setting a rule that only one person talks at once. When family and friends know the reason for these rules, they will usually be glad to follow them. Here are some suggestions for routines:

Have a weekly guys (or gals) afternoon. The PwLBD and two or three close friends/family can meet for cards or something else enjoyable. Besides providing an afternoon of sociability, this frees the care partner for a few hours of needed respite. The PwLBD will feel most comfortable if the group meets at your home.

Invite a friend in. Arrange for a friend to visit the PwLBD for a couple of hours each week. The two can play cards or board games, talk or even read aloud—whatever sounds fun. While this sounds similar to the previous suggestion, it isn't. As the disorder advances, even small groups may become too stressful but a single visitor will still be enjoyable.

Go on a weekly outing with friends/family. Arrange for the PwLBD to go with friends on a short weekly outing to play golf, to eat out, to….. It should be the same activity every time. The sameness promotes comfort. Besides, variety loses its attraction very quickly for anyone who is facing dementia.

Enjoy a child. Invite a grandchild or neighbor child to visit on a regular basis. (Remember the one-at-a-time rule; more can be overwhelming.) Help the PwLBD to start an ongoing project with the child's help: putting photos in an album or scrapbooking or even gardening. Both PwLB and child will have fun and may develop a special rapport that will continue to be a blessing as the disorder advances.

Children often have a special ability to connect. They have fewer expectations and accept people at face value. However, as children grow into teenagers, that can change. Some can be very helpful while others are too busy dealing with their own issues. Plan projects together with the PwLB.

Exercise with family or friends. Encourage the PwLBD to go swimming, play tennis, or participate in any other sport he enjoys. Consider joining him and making it a team activity. After all, care partners need exercise too.

Routines involving friends and family set up a win-win situation. They help the PwLBD fight dementia by enjoying a social visit or an outing with valued friends/family. At the same time, they provide the care partner with valuable time to experience a few hours of respite.

Chapter 43

Community and Internet Support

Communities offer a variety of support besides those focusing specifically on Lewy body disorders.

Groups and Organizations

Does your loved one already belong to a group? Bridge, golfing, dancing and tennis have already been mentioned. Maybe he belongs to a lodge, a professional organization, or church group. Even when he can no longer do the activity, the PwLBD may be able to participate. Dean's tennis group (See Chapter 29.) invited him to come watch their matches and join in their social hours. The PwLB's group may not think to include him unless asked to do so. Reach out to see what each has to offer. Sometimes, what the group offers won't be connected with the group's main activity. When Joan stopped playing bridge (See Chapter 32), group members didn't encourage her to return; the game was beyond her. Instead, some of the members kept Joan company while her daughter went shopping.

Community Support

Many community groups can provide help for a Lewy team. Besides Parkinson's and Alzheimer's organizations, there are many others: senior centers, community colleges with classes for seniors, Meals on Wheels or other food services. Start with the local Area Agency on Aging which can suggest others. Each organization has its place and use. Look for:

Information. What does the group know about LB disorders and the issues involved?

Ease of Access. Is the location close by? If not, is there a similar group closer to you? Or can you access information and services via phone or internet?

Services. What dementia and senior related services does the organization offer, such as support groups, a health library, classes, meals, tax preparation, free legal consultations or referrals to other helpful agencies?

Internet Support

It may be difficult to find adequate information or support in person. Therefore, the internet is a resource that every LBD family should utilize. If you don't have a computer or internet connection, libraries have computers to use. If you are not computer-literate, develop some basic skills or find someone who will help. The information and support available via the internet for both members of the Lewy team is enormous.

Besides the LBDA website and our own website, LBDtools.com, there are many other internet resources with great information and internet stores with products for families dealing with Lewy body disorders. Many are listed in the Resources section of this book.

Section Eight:

A Lewy-Friendly Home

When is it time to consider assisted living? Many caregivers believe that it is when coping at home is no longer possible. "Not," they say, "while my loved one is still functional and the care partner is in good health." Wrong! This IS the time to consider such changes and plan ahead. Early on, it is easier to make still difficult decisions and act upon them.

Each Lewy team has these decisions, with their own solutions. Some decide by not deciding—by staying where they are as long as they can and letting the disorder decide for them. Others take control of the situation and start making decisions early on. These people are the ones who will usually have the least stress.

Plans make things go smoother. If you decide to keep the PwLBD at home, remodeling will likely be needed. If you want move to a more accessible home or if you decide on assisted living, searching out just the right place takes time.

Be aware that research has shown that DLB patients, with physical problems involving the autonomic nervous system and drug sensitivity, tend to require the use of more resources than those with Alzheimer's.[111] This means that a move to assisted living or to round-the-clock home care might be necessary much sooner than expected. If the PwLBD also has Parkinson's, then the additional mobility issues will likely be even more demanding and the move could be even sooner.

Chapter 44

Decisions About Where to Live

Lewy teams often promise each other that the PwLBD can always stay in their home. It may seem an easy promise at first.

> *Early on, Del and I talked about our future. He begged me not to put him in a nursing home. It was easy to agree. I didn't want that for him either. But I began to see that the time might come when I'd have to consider a residential placement. That's when I started answering Del's pleas, "I will keep you here as long as I possibly can." -- Nancy*

Eventually, Nancy realized that caring for Del at home had become unsafe. LBD does not stand still. The PwLB develops more symptoms, becomes more physically impaired and moves continually closer to dementia. The care partner changes too, with issues and illnesses that limit their abilities or may even be life threatening. Planning for these possible changes before they happen and making decisions as a team can decrease the problems and make the ones that do occur less painful.

There are three main reasons that people with dementia end up in long term care:

The PwLB's declining abilities or health. The PwLB's failing health is the first reason that usually comes to mind. Due to the increased physical issues that accompany Lewy body dementia, PwLBD often need long term care sooner than someone with Alzheimer's or another type of dementia.[112] In addition, a person with LBD is more likely than someone with Alzheimer's to have coexisting illnesses. Depression is certainly one of these, but so are migraines and strokes. Strokes especially, may make living at home more difficult.[113]

Two other reasons are also common.

Lack of accessibility. When people require help to get around, things change, living space needs change. There are a multitude of things a Lewy team may not even consider until not having them makes life difficult. Of course, PwPDD, the type of LBD that starts out with Parkinson's are most likely to fit this category.

Caregiver illness. More PwLB go into long-term care due to the caregiver's poor health than due to their own illnesses. With 24/7 responsibilities, continual lifting and bending, caregiver stress and bad backs are too often the norm. The care partner's body rebels in other ways as well, with heart problems, diabetes, or a variety of illnesses.[114]

Warning: Dementia caregiving, even in a handicap-accessible home, is not a one-person job. Trying to do this alone is a setup for caregiver illness, the number one reason for long term care.

Be sure to include funds for adequate help in your planning. Home care may be as expensive, or even more expensive than residential care.

In addition to the physical stresses, LBD caregivers experience the isolation related to dementia caregiving in general, the emotional stress related to dealing with their loved one's ongoing acting-out behaviors and the feeling that others don't understand these issues well enough to help. This added stress decreases the caregiver's ability to deal with physical issues, resulting in even more physical problems.

Accessibility

A more accessible home decreases the dangers to a care partner's health while allowing the PwLB to stay home longer. Plan for better accessibility in these ways:

Remodel the present home

Advantages: The stress of leaving a familiar home is avoided or at least, moved further into the future.

Concern: Remodeling can be expensive initially.

Helpful hint: Renovations can often be off-set with an increased home valuation.

Concern: Remodeling can also be stressful, with strangers in the home and all the changes.

Helpful hint: Do any remodeling early in the LB journey while cognitive functioning is good most of the time.

Concern: With LBD's relentless degeneration, round-the-clock care will likely be required sooner rather than later.

Helpful hint: If round-the-clock care will not be financially feasible, seriously consider assisted living instead of major remodeling.

Move to a more accessible, usually smaller home

Advantages: The Lewy team can still live at home with familiar furniture and belongings.

Concern: Moving can be expensive and entails a major change. The stress of leaving a place where the PwLBD has lived for a long time can be extreme, especially when done well into the LB journey when change is difficult.

Helpful hint: The earlier you can make this move, the better.

Helpful hint: Such an event, where stress is to be expected, is one of the few times when a preventative short regimen of a mild, quick-acting behavior management drug might be helpful. This may avert the need for more, stronger drugs later.

Concern: As with remodeling, a move to assisted living may still be required eventually, with the second move made after the PwLBD is less able to tolerate change.

Helpful hint: If round-the-clock home care will not be financially or otherwise feasible when needed, consider making a single move to assisted living.

Move into assisted living

Advantages: Someone else takes over the physical caregiving. This allows the care partner to focus on being a partner/spouse instead of so much on household and caregiver chores.

Concern: This is usually a very frightening choice for the PwLBD because they fear being abandoned to the care of strangers in a strange place.

Helpful hint: Sometimes the care partner can move into an assisted living facility along with the PwLB. This can decrease both the fear of abandonment and feelings of guilt. If that isn't practical, the care partner can plan to spend much of the day in the facility at first so as to limit this fear.

Helpful hint: As with moving into a smaller place, this is another time when a short regimen of a low dose, short-acting behavior management drug might avert the need for more, stronger drugs later.

Helpful hint: PwLBD will often start asking to "go home" when they feel tired. Take this as time for you to say "I'm going to step out for a while so that you can take a nap." (Don't say "good by"..that may be too scary.)

Chapter 45

Staying At Home

Most Lewy teams will decide to stay at home at first. There are many ways to make a home Lewy-friendlier. Remodeling can be expensive but very helpful. Some teams may choose to downsize and move to a smaller place that is already handicap accessible. There are also many less expensive ways to make a home safer.

Is Staying at Home Practical?

Naturally this is a personal decision for each Lewy team. The first thing to consider is if staying at home will be practical. If long term care will eventually be required anyway, then major renovations or other changes may not be the way to go. Of course, the less expensive, often temporary changes are still viable.

LBD is a debilitating disorder. If the PwLBD has the kind that starts with Parkinson's, it is most debilitating but even DLB causes more problems than other dementias such as Alzheimer's. Thus any consideration for staying at home must also include the financial cost of eventual round-the-clock home care by experienced staff. If this is not possible, then planning for long term home care is probably not practical.

When mobility isn't an issue, as it often isn't with DLB, other issues may be equally concerning.

Annie was physically able to walk and take care of her daily living activities. I never thought the time would come when I couldn't take care of her at home. But it did. She became very combative and no matter what I did, I couldn't change that. When I took her to the ER because I didn't know what else to do, Social Services stepped in and made the decision for me. – Jim Whitworth

That was in the early 2002. We know a lot more about dealing with LBD's acting-out behaviors now. Better caregiver education and a variety of drugs and traditional therapies can reduce the acting-out behavior like Annie's, but there will usually still be some. If the caregiver is not able to deal with these in a way that is supportive to both caregiver and loved one, then long term home care is not practical.

Remodeling

In her book, *Treasures in the Darkness*, Pat Snyder[115] shares that when she and John remodeled, they hoped the improvements would allow him to stay home longer. They did; six years later, he was still at home. Renovations can be expensive. However, such home improvements will usually increase the sales value of a home. In addition, Pat reports that their costs were offset and more by the lower cost of living at home vs. the cost of residential care. When comparing these figures, don't forget to include the expense of eventual round-the-clock help, which can be needed well before the end of the Lewy journey. These costs will depend on your area, and may actually make home care more expensive than residential care.

During the remodel planning phase, plan for as many physical and cognitive problems as possible. Think carefully about what you will need in the future and plan for these eventualities even if the equipment isn't needed now. Later installation of special equipment will usually be more difficult and more expensive as well.

Ask for an in-home OT evaluation. An occupational therapist can be very helpful in advising on the changes needed. The therapist may also have information about getting insurance coverage for the changes.

Replace entry steps with a ramp. An attractive entryway and ramp can add value to a house. Ramps are easier for an unsteady walker to negotiate and if a wheelchair is ever needed, the transition will be easier. A ramp narrow enough to allow a person to use railings on both sides but wide enough for a wheelchair is optimal. Make sure there is at least one usable railing if the ramp is wider.

Make a sanctuary area where the care partner can relax undisturbed. Care partner "downtime" is a great stress reliever—for both members of the team. While you can arrange for this at any time, adding it to the remodeling plans will make it more likely to happen. Use a secluded area: a spare room, or a quiet corner away from the action. A recliner chair for relaxing and reading so that you can do your research comfortably is a priority. So is a computer for access to online groups so that you can easily reach out to others in times of stress. Add anything else that will make this a pleasant place for you to wind down.

Replace door knobs with pull handles or levers. These are easier for Lewy-damaged hands to grasp and use.

Cover mirrors with something you can open as needed. A person with dementia-damaged perceptions may see a stranger in the mirror instead of his own image and be frightened.

Remove unneeded mirrors. Add swinging shutters, pull-back drapes or pull-up shades to those you want to keep.

In the bathroom, consider the following:

Install grab bars near toilet and bathing areas to prevent falls and aid independence. Make sure the bar surface is lightly textured to prevent slipping.

Make all or most of the room an open "wet area." Easier access and cleanup can save hours of frustration and work when there is only a curtain and no floor barrier between the shower and the rest of the room.

Position the drain so that the floor slopes very gradually, perhaps towards one corner instead of the middle of the area. This provides better footing and less chance of falling.

Install a shower hose so that it easily reaches the toileting area, making cleanup much simpler.

Place a heat lamp with a timer in the ceiling to warm the bathroom safely. PwLBD who have lost the ability to verbalize their discomfort tend to avoid a cold bathroom. Avoid dangerous portable space heaters.

Remove the door locks. As confusion sets in, the PwLBD may lock the bathroom door but not be able to unlock it. Install a keypad lock if one is needed for other members of the family.

Install doors that open out to prevent the PwLBD from blocking the door with his body if he falls in the bathroom. This grows in importance as he becomes less able to follow instructions.

Put up open shelves for needed items like towels and toilet paper. Having such supplies out in plain sight and easily accessible increases independence and avoids confusion.

Hide electrical outlets in lockable cupboards. This keeps the outlets accessible for use now. When and if judgment disappears, the outlets will be out of reach.

Don't depend on the new tamper-resistant outlets. These are great for preventing children from getting shocked. However, the concern is different for an adult. The PwLBD is much more likely to use the outlet properly to run an unsafe appliance.

Some Less Expensive Ideas

Whether you can remodel or not, these following suggestions cost very little and can make a home much more Lewy-friendly. Susan Scarff offers many more in her book, *Dementia, The Journey Ahead.*[116]

Use sheets for mirror covers. Sheets make good mirror covers if you don't want to go to the trouble of removing the mirrors or making a more elaborate cover. It is also fairly easy to put up a curtain rod and hang curtains over the mirrors.

Use keyed locks for outside doors and those to the garage or anyplace with dangerous equipment. As with the locked bathroom cabinets, the PwLB will be able to access these areas now but the locks can become active when the ability to identify danger decreases. An alarm that sounds when a door opens adds to safety.

Use interlocking foam mats to cover the bathroom floor. These can be picked up and cleaned in the shower. They also cushion falls.

Make walking paths in the house that are straight, direct and as free from furniture as possible to reduce confusion and falling.

Simplify and remove unnecessary clutter. Remove unnecessary furniture. This is both a focus issue and a safety issue. Open space is less confusing and easier to navigate without falling.

Remove area rugs. Rugs may soften a fall, but can also cause accidents when an already unsteady person trips over a rumpled edge.

Pad sharp corners and edges. Swimming noodles cut in sections work well for this.

Lower the hot water temperature to 110 degrees or less to avoid burns. Most dishwashers have an internal water heater and most laundry detergents now do a fine job with cold or warm water. Hotter temperatures aren't needed.

Use good, but soft non-glare, lighting. This reduces the dark areas and shadows that can cause confusion yet provides the light needed to avoid falls and bumping into the furniture. Keep some lights on in the bathroom even at night to limit confusion during nocturnal bathroom trips.

Consider padding the PwLB's bedroom floor or at least the area by the bed. As LBD advances, a couple of issues make falls in bedrooms especially common. Active Dreams can cause the PwLBD to move around so much that he falls out of bed. (See

Chapter 6.) Falls from orthostatic hypotension (low blood pressure on rising), can also occur early in the LB journey. (See Chapter 8.)

> *I have Active Dreams. They don't bother me except that once in a while, I fall out of bed. Joyce got worried that I'd hurt myself. Her support group suggested those interlocking mats used in garages. I wasn't all that excited about it but she found some in green that don't look too garish and so I agreed to try them. It took me a couple of days to lay the squares. It would only have taken me a couple of hours to do the job a few years ago, but at least I was still able to do it! And hey! They work. I still fall out of bed now and then, but no more bruises! — Phil*

Rubber tumbling mats might work even better for around the bed. They come in a multitude of sizes and thicknesses. Be aware that the softer the pad, the more difficult it will be to walk on and maintain one's balance.

Use pressure monitors, which alert the care partner when the PwLBD gets up from bed at night. He is often at his most confused then and may not know he needs help, or be able to ask for it even if he does.

> *Dad wakes up at night and tries to get up by himself. Invariably he falls if I don't get to him soon enough. I tried a baby monitor and it worked as long as I was awake but I needed more. Then we got a pressure monitor. Dad and I both like this. It sounds an alarm as soon as he starts to get up so that I can get there before he falls. We also use one in his*

chair. He's always forgetting to call me when he wants to get out of it. — Doris

Doris had her alarm in her bedroom so that she could hear it. Phil, who has Active Dreams, might want his nearby so it would warn him before he fell out of bed.

Use a bedside commode. If there is room, consider placing a commode near the bed so the PwLBD doesn't have to travel so far. This can limit confusion too.

Moving to a Different Place

Some Lewy teams have homes that aren't right for the kind of remodeling needed to make a home Lewy-friendly. Other teams would rather move than remodel.

When considering a smaller home, remember that round-the-clock care will likely be an eventual necessity. If this isn't financially or otherwise possible in the home, any move to a smaller, more accessible place should be considered very early in the progress of the disorder, ideally even before any evidence of cognitive degeneration is present.

If you choose to move, start by deciding what criteria is important. At the least, it should include:

- Doorways and bathrooms big enough for wheelchairs.
- Street level entryways (or ramps).
- Everything on one floor.
- Bathrooms with grab bars and high toilets.
- Size and floor plan that is easy for the care partner to manage.

Many of suggestions in the section on remodeling may also very helpful.

Start this process as early as possible. Some care partners have benefited from their experiences with their PwLBD and have started this process themselves while still in quite good health.

I own a small apartment house. One of the apartments is already handicap accessible. Now that Bud is gone, I'm fixing it up for me so that when I can no longer live in this big house with so many stairs, I can move there. It is right in town, close to bus routes and stores. I won't even need a car to get around. My daughter lives close by too. — Jo

Due to her experience as a care partner, Jo already has a good idea of what is needed. For instance, she knows that even though she can drive and negotiate stairs easily now, it may not always be that way. She wants family support and so she is making it easy for that to happen.

We know the time is coming when Dad will need to move into something safer and easier to get around than his house. He isn't crazy about moving but he does like the idea of being close to us. We are remodeling the garage into a studio apartment so Dad can be close but independent as well. — Rosemary

Jo and Rosemary are both making plans now for what will be needed in the future. This will make the move much less traumatic. When dementia is involved, start the planning even before the need shows up. Make the move before your loved one has lost the ability to adapt. This will almost always be well before the change is a physical necessity.

Chapter 46

Long Term Care

Moving into long term care (LTC) is something that most Lewy teams prefer to consider only as a last resort. However, it might be a better choice than it initially seems. As with living at home, there are several choices. Assisted living offers a lot of independence. An adult family home feels more family-like and is less distracting. For someone with LBD, a locked memory care facility may not be needed until much later, if at all. However, in each case, staff who are comfortable working with people with dementia is a must.

Assisted Living

An assisted living (AL) facility differs from a memory unit in that it houses residents with a variety of problems besides dementia. Memory care units are usually locked to prevent wandering, which is seldom an issue with Lewy body dementia (unless, of course the person also has Alzheimer's). Many PwLBD can stay in assisted living even with well advanced dementia.

AL offers some independence with residents providing some of their own self-care. Each unit is a small suite that includes a kitchen and bathroom. There's physical and medical support available as needed and at least one prepared meal a day.

Some AL facilities encourage caregivers to live there with their loved ones for only the cost of the food they eat. This may seem odd, but it benefits the facility. Residents are happier and get better care with less staff time required.

Bud was sitting in our big leather chair and I was sitting on his lap. We were talking about the assisted living place we'd been to see. "We can do it," I said. Bud nodded. "We can do it," he agreed. We had to wait for a room to come open and when it did months later, we were in our winter home, a thousand miles away. Rather than pack up and leave, we decided to wait for the next opening. Bud was doing fine. He didn't need that much care yet, we told each other. — Jo

Later, Jo and Bud changed their mind and decided to remodel their big family home instead of entering assisted living.

That was a mistake. We loved our home but it wasn't right for the kind of remodeling Bud needed. Too many stairs, a bathroom that was far too small, and a multitude of other things we couldn't change. In hindsight, I so wish we'd made that difficult move to assisted living while we could still adapt and make it our home. — Jo

Reasons for an Early Move to LTC

There are several reasons to consider an assisted living situation early in the Lewy journey.

Better adjustment. Perhaps the most unlikely reason for considering assisted living is also the best reason. Most care partners say they want to keep their loved one at home as long as they can. However, the more thinking ability a PwLB has when he enter a long term facility, the better he will adjust.

A person with only mild dementia can still adjust to new spaces, make new friends and participate in activities. Such a person also will have more insight and will be better able to understand the need for the move. A person admitted with full-blown dementia will sit in a chair in a room and vegetate. He can't—and it is *can't*, not *won't*—adapt. The advantage for the care partner is equally great. Your health will be better, with more energy and time. It is not unusual for relationships to improve when the physical responsibilities are in someone else's hands.

> *I put off placing Del into a care facility. I felt guilty even considering it. But the time came when I felt I had no choice. Now I wish I'd done it sooner. I was still with Del every day, but I went home in the evening and actually slept well at night and so I was more rested—and patient. With the staff doing all the heavy lifting and hard work, my role became one of wife and companion again. We both loved the change.*
> — *Nancy*

Don't let pleas or guilt deprive the Lewy team of the improved life that an early move into assisted living can often provide. Don't wait until the PwLB wants to go. No one is going to say "I want to leave my familiar home and move to someplace where strangers will be in my business." Don't wait until you feel there's no other choice. By then, it is usually well past time. When there's a chance of long term care in future, consider it earlier rather than later.

Safety. Dementia may cause a PwLBD to be unable to recognize a dangerous situation even while still appearing—and feeling—fully functional. When this is the case, a person can no more be left alone than could an active preschooler.

> *I work fulltime and Roy stays home by himself. So far, this has gone well. He doesn't try to cook or anything like that.*

But sometimes, he sure can make a mess. Last week I came home to find that he'd disassembled the kitchen light switch. "It wasn't working right," he told me. He was an electrician and so this should have been a piece of cake for him. But he hadn't been able to get it back together and so now I don't have a light in the kitchen and I'm going to have to hire someone to come fix it. — Sharon

Sharon may need to rethink her statement about Roy's safety. He could have electrocuted himself if he had tried to work on the light switch without first turning off the electricity. The awareness of the need for safety precautions requires the ability to understand cause and effect, which can go before task abilities do. If adequate supervision is unavailable at home, this is a good reason for residential care, or at the very least adult day care.

Difficult early symptoms. Behavioral symptoms may show up early and be difficult for the care partner to deal with. There may be poor eating or drinking, leading to an increase of other Lewy symptoms, including acting-out. Sometimes, symptoms such as delusions can result in violence or threats of violence. When this occurs, it becomes a safety issue and the Lewy team may have to consider residential care, with staff that is trained to deal with these kinds of issues.

I'm at my wit's end. Larry was diagnosed with LBD only six months ago. I thought we'd have a few years at least before things got bad. But I can't believe it. Larry is peeing everywhere. In a flower pot, on the sofa, in the garbage can, in the closet. I'm worn out trying to clean up all of his messes. I tried signs, even picture signs but that didn't work. I set up a schedule and take him to the toilet every two hours. He just stands there. And then fifteen minutes later, he's peeing against the wall in the bedroom. I tried to make him wear diapers, but he takes them off. I just don't know what to do next. — Doris

Larry's LBD-caused impulsiveness has overcome the social skills he learned as a child. Each case is different. Sometimes this happens very early in the disorder and sometimes it might not happen at all. Some caregivers might be able to deal with Larry's behavior even if they couldn't keep it from happening. However, it is causing Doris major stress, which likely makes Larry's behavior even worse.

The caregiver's health must be a primary consideration. High stress leads to poor health, which often results in an eventual inability to do the job well, if at all. Once Doris has exhausted all her ideas without adequate result, it may be time for her to consider residential care where others, likely younger and more experienced, can deal with Larry's lack of inhibition.

The PwLB's health and abilities. Health issues that cannot be addressed well at home become very good reasons for residential care. Repeated episodes of dehydration, lifting that the care partner can't do safely, or inadequate nutrition might all be reasons to consider LTC.

I have diabetes as well as MCI. I can get around fine and I can even drive but I knew I wasn't eating right. I decided to move into an assisted living facility so that I could get a better diet. I love it. I only cook when I want to now and yet I'm eating much better than I used to. There are many activities to keep me busy too. I'm much happier here than I was in my little apartment. And if I need more care, it's in a different part of the same building. – Edith

Edith lived alone and knew she needed better care than she was providing for herself. Incidentally, she also found that she loved the socializing that was so easy there.

If you wait until the health issues are severe, the PwLBD may need more care than assisted living provides. This is a huge incentive for considering a move while the PwLBD is still physically and mentally functional.

The care partner's health. In Chapter 44, Nancy tells how she promised Del she'd keep him at home as long as she possibly could. Like many care partners, Nancy hadn't considered her own health when she made that promise. "As long as it is safe for both of us" is a better answer. When coping becomes difficult, the PwLBD mirrors your stress and symptoms increase. This makes an already overwhelming job even more troublesome and caregiver illness more likely.

In addition, the PwLBD may not be getting the care he needs. When your health and stamina are gone, there will no longer be a choice. Residential placement will be the only answer. The problem is that by then, the PwLB's condition may have progressed to where adjustment to the move is impossible.

Adult Family Homes

An adult family home may be a better choice for the PwLBD than a large assisted living facility, even if the care partner can visit often. The variety of activities and free family access that make an assisted living program attractive to the family may not be helpful for the PwLBD.

We spent weeks looking for just the right place for Dad. We finally settled on one that was close enough so that I could visit easily and big enough that it had lots of activities. Best of all, the staff was supportive and loving. At first Dad did fine, but as his LBD got worse, he became belligerent and angry. I could see the problem. He needed less stimulation. The activities that were so attractive had become frustrating and bothersome. The comings and goings of the residents' families surrounded him with strangers and too much noise. He always liked walking when he was upset and he started leaving the facility to take walks. When the staff tried to stop him, he felt attacked and struck out. I had to find another place. This time, I chose a small group home with only four other residents. Dad is doing well there. — Joy Walker[117]

Joy had done her homework and found what she thought was the perfect place for her dad. She had assumed he'd be able to stay there for the rest of his life. The continual bustle of activity and noise that was initially attractive to Joy was overwhelming to her dad and he communicated this by his behavior.

When PwLBD must enter long term care alone, the teams usually wait longer to consider placement.

I knew that Mom would probably adjust better if we placed her in assisted living sooner, but I just couldn't do it. We were doing fine and I wanted her to be able to stay in her own home just as long as she could. But eventually, I realized that she needed more than I could provide at home. By then, I didn't think Mom would do well in assisted living. Instead, I found a nice group home for her and after a few weeks of adjustment, she actually likes it. — Janet

Adult family homes worked better for Joy's dad and Janet's mom for the following reasons:

- LBD had already decreased their ability to adapt. With fewer staff, residents and space, adapting was easier.
- Dementia had also made them sensitive to extremes—noise, crowd and even the bustle of activities. A smaller home with fewer activities was less stimulating.

There still needs to be a caring, supportive staff. It helps if the staff is also Lewy-savvy and non-drug oriented. The downside of group homes is that staff may be less well trained. Check this out carefully. Because adapting tends to be easier, choosing a group home may extend the time at home. However, the issues remain. Waiting still decreases the PwLB's ability to adapt and the care partner's chance of illness while increasing safety concerns. Don't wait too long!

Affording Residential Care

Residential care is never cheap. The section on Funding Sources in Chapter 17 offers some suggestions for obtaining financial help. The Resource Section provides the names of some agencies and programs that offer assistance.

Insurance. Most regular insurance plans do not include residential placement except for rehabilitation and then for only short periods of time. Long term care (LTC) insurance is expensive, but worth buying—*if it is done before the PwLB is diagnosed with any kind of dementia.* Afterward, the cost will be prohibitive. Also see Chapter 17 for other issues to consider when buying this insurance.

At-Home Care. An alternative to residential care is round-the-clock in-home help. Most Lewy teams start with in-home help a few hours a week, adding more hours as needed. However, when the time comes for round-the clock care, residential placement may be less expensive. Depending on the in-home help available and affordable, residential placement may also provide better care. Finally, by then it may also be the best solution for the care partner's health.

Some teams may try to get by with only a small amount of outside care. This is a mistake. At the stage where the PwLBD needs the kind of care a residential facility provides, home care staff should be round-the-clock. The care partner will still be there 24/7 as care manager, companion, advocate and support person. Adding exhausting physical tasks or sleepless nights may be enough to push one over the edge and residential care will be needed anyway.

Adult Day Care

Many long term care communities offer adult day care (ADC), where the PwLBD spends several hours a day several days a week with other seniors. Such a program can provide some respite for the care partner and lengthen the time before residential care may be needed. If the care partner works, this may be a better choice than in-home help--and it may be less expensive. Transportation is usually provided.

The place that sponsors my support group offers free day care for loved ones during our monthly meetings and Bobby usually goes. Lately, my group has been warning me that I need more help. Even though I knew they were right, in-home care doesn't work for us. Instead, I've started taking Bobby to day care once a week. I especially like that I can arrange for the staff to give him his bath on the day he goes. It's worth the extra fee because bathing him has really become difficult for me. He's still ambivalent—some days he likes it and some days he doesn't but I've been adamant. I tell him I need this to keep my health. My goal is actually full residential care in a few months. -- Marlene

Many residential facilities offer free care for support group member's loved ones during the meeting. If you choose to utilize regular day care, be sure to check on extra services such as bathing. This may extend the time you will be able to safely keep the PwLBD at home.

Marlene is using Adult Day Care as a stepping stone to residential, so that both she and her husband can become used to the change more gradually. Like Bobby, most PwLBD will be resistive. This is when a care partner must be strong and stick with what they know is best in the long run.

Roger goes to the Adult Day Club twice a week. He was hesitant first but now he loves it. I started having him go so I could get a break, but now, he's standing by the door waiting impatiently for the buss that transports him. -- Ella

Adult day care can provide socialization for the PwLBD who seldom gets out anymore. As with residential care, it is a good idea to start these visits long before they are needed.

See the *Guide*, page 175 for more about this choice.

The Right Place

Here are the main things to look for when choosing a long term care program:

- The staff is familiar with LBD, its fluctuations and its drug issues.
- The focus is on behavior management techniques first and drugs for behavior only when the non-drug tools aren't adequate. Such a place may be more expensive. The more behavior management drugs a facility uses, the fewer staff is usually required.
- Staff treats the PwLBD with care and respect.
- Staff and administration view the care partner as part of the team.

For more suggestions about what to look for, go to Chapter 12 in the *Guide*, page 188.

Socialization Issues in Residential Care

Once the move is made, the care partner has a whole new set of responsibilities. (See the *Guide*, pages 192-195.) With someone else responsible for physical care, you can focus on the PwLB's emotional wellbeing—and on maintaining the relationship that the two of you have enjoyed for years.

Staff members are very good at providing physical care but not so good at being social. They just don't have the time. Residents tend to have fewer casual interactions and more instances where they are "talked at" during caregiving or in leader-centered group discussions. Such one-way transactions do not meet a PwLB's need for socialization, and he will begin to lose the skills he still has. It is up to the care partner, family and friends to provide adequate socialization, that is, two-way conversations about something other than daily care.

Hold conversations, visit, and enjoy each other. This is not a minor thing. It isn't just useless small talk. When the PwLBD feels encouraged to talk, communication lasts longer with less frustration.

Relax together. With someone else taking care of the physical requirements, the care partner will be less tired, overwhelmed and stressed. The PwLBD will mirror this and relax more too.

Use visual aids like picture albums or scrapbooks to trigger thoughts and provide something to talk about. Ask questions. Listen to the stories.

Visit on a regular basis. If the care partner does not live in the facility, time visits for when the PwLBD is at their best. Unless you help with daily chores like dressing, come when these tasks are done.

Summary

- PwLBD tend to need 24/7 care sooner than those with other dementias, due to physical disabilities and illnesses.
- Home care is only practical if adequate help is available and affordable. This eventually means round-the-clock staffing.
- More people enter residential care because of their caregiver's ill health than because of their own.

- People who enter residential care after their ability to socialize is compromised do not do as well as those who enter while that ability is still at least partially intact.
- Some Assisted Living facilities allow their resident's spouses to live with them for only the price of the meals they eat.
- Adult Family Homes may offer less stimulation and the person with more advanced dementia may find it easier to adapt to their smaller environment.
- Utilizing Adult Day Care may offer a less expensive way to provide necessary supervision, thus extending the time before residential care is required. It also provides socialization.
- Socialization is an important part of the care partner's job, in or out of a care facility.

Section Nine:

Getting On With Life

Especially if the PwLBD already has Parkinson's, you know it isn't the end of the world. You still have lives to live. You may have to adjust and adapt, but there are still things to do, places to go, people to see. There are still family and friends. There are still hobbies although they may be a bit different now—more limited, perhaps, but still there. For instance, The PwPD may do workouts at the gym instead of jogging or tend house plants instead of a garden.

It's the same for LBD. As cognitive abilities decline, the team must adapt and change to meet these challenges. Don't give up. Staying active adds oxygen and stimulates the brain, both of which are needed to maintain quality of life and independence while pushing dependence further into the future.

Chapter 47

Adapting Without Giving Up

Eventually, most activities will become more difficult for the PwLB. As long as safety isn't involved, quitting isn't necessary. With a change of perspective, some pre-planning and the help of family and friends, he should be able to continue many enjoyable pursuits.

Change the goal from "excelling" to "persevering." As people age, it is natural to become less proficient than in the past. The decline is simply quicker when dementia is involved. Where once the challenge was to improve, now it is to continue.

Give credit. Encourage the PwLB to give himself credit for tenacity and hard work. With LBD, nothing is second nature and every move must be contemplated. Simply continuing to do a beloved activity takes at least as much effort as excelling at the same activity used to take.

Adapt. When the PwLBD can't do an activity any longer, help him find a way to adapt it so that he can. If he plays tennis, maybe he can move closer to the net. Help a scrap booker find simpler motifs or a card player a simpler game. Eventually, the new form may become too difficult too. Adapt again. And again. The goal is to keep active, keep busy, and keep on using the brain.

Offer and accept help. As activities become harder to do, care partners or others may be able to provide support. Part of the care partner's job is to help the your loved one accept other's help while maintaining dignity.

We've square danced for years and even after Maxie had difficulty remembering the moves, we continued to dance. Our square-mates generously helped her and we all had fun. — Burt

Offering help matter-of-factly and with a smile is makes it easier for the PwLBD to accept. Judy Jennings talked in her book about doing crossword puzzles as a team when Dean could no longer do them alone. Judy's obvious enjoyment of the activity made it easier for Dean to accept her help.

Help the PwLB prepare for letting go of unsafe tasks. Think now about how to know when such things as driving, using a check book, or cooking have become unsafe. Letting go of tasks like these that help to define a person as an adult is never easy. Do what you can to help HIM be the one to decide to let these go. It will be much less traumatic than if someone else makes decision for him.

That said, your job as a team is to get on with life. Charles Schneider[118] says it this way in his book, *Don't Bury Me, It Ain't Over Yet:*

Even though we are slow and not capable of everything we used to be able to do, we still want to . . . contribute in every way we can. It's easy to get so wrapped up in our problems that we forget the most precious things, sharing, loving and laughing. We don't want to be excluded.

What's on your Lewy team's "bucket list?" Charles Schneider made a list of ventures he wanted to complete before he "faded away." Among other things, Charles wanted to take his grandson fishing—and he did. What would be on your list? Travel? Reading a special book? Finishing a project?

Don't forget to include present activities. Dean Jennings wanted to continue to play tennis and so he worked to be able to do that. Coy wanted to continue playing golf. Which of the the PwLBD's present interests are important enough to merit the hard work required to continue doing it?

Maintain the connection with family and friends. As a LB disorder progresses, it can take away the ability to show expression and even talk, which makes this task more complicated. Isolation becomes easier for the loved one than reaching out. As responsibilities pile up, isolation also becomes an issue for the care partner. Start early, while it is easier and there is more time, to let people know how important they are to your team.

Chapter 48

Travel

Travel often tops a PwLB's bucket list.

> *Chuck had two wishes: to see the Grand Canyon and to attend a baseball spring training game. Since both are in Arizona, we did it all in one trip. I made the arrangements ahead of time and thank goodness, it all went smoothly. Chuck's favorite team won all three of the games we watched and so we considered the trip worth the effort. — Florrie Munat, in her book, Be Brave.*

A long trip takes lot of effort and planning when someone with LBD is involved. Making a long journey wasn't something Chuck and Florrie did on a whim. Florrie prepared for the above trip carefully.

Care partners often wonder if it is too late for them to travel.

> *My husband, Dwight, wants to fly across the country to visit family in his home town one more time this summer. He's just been diagnosed with LBD but we've seen symptoms for a couple of years. He's still very functional and but he has quit driving and he can get confused easily. Should he go? I'm working but I can take the time off if I have to. Should I go with him? —Lorna*

Many people with mild LBD travel and do fine. Plan ahead, keep the stress down, and always go with a care partner. Jim and Annie flew to Europe. Judy and Dean Jennings also traveled to Europe several times. The *Guide* tells how Barbara and Bill

Hutchinson took an RV from Alaska to Florida. It can be done—but if Dwight decides to go, they shouldn't wait. The longer they put it off, the more problems there will be.

Don't let a person with even mild dementia go alone. The first task when planning a trip is to decide who is going. Lorna should definitely go with Dwight. PwLBD should *never* travel alone. Even with those who feel very able to do so, the disorder fluctuates greatly. Low levels can appear just when clarity is needed most—when the stress is at its worst. Someone must go along to assist during the rough spots. Assure the PwLBD that this is being smart, not helpless.

Plan, plan, plan. The more you plan, the fewer surprises, the less stress. Plan ways to avoid extremes and add familiarity and comfort. If going by car, plan short trips to avoid tiredness (probably no more than two or at most three hundred miles a day). Pack extra clothes for warmth. Take known routes whenever possible. Consider emergencies that might come up and how to deal with them. Talk to the doctor about extra medications.

Do the nitty-gritty stuff. Even when the PwLBD is functioning well, the truth is that you will probably have to do most of the planning and initiating. Remember what Charles Schneider said about challenges in Chapter 29. Once dementia is present, the challenge is no longer making things happen but simply to keep doing.

Plan as a team. This may sound like a contradiction to the above. It isn't. Yes, you will take on the responsibility for making sure everything runs smoothly. But make sure the PwLBD doesn't opt out of the planning altogether. Encourage him to be involved and to be in on the decisions. Even if he forgets the details, his sense of involvement will remain. He will feel more in control. The trip will be less stressful—and more fun for both of you.

Keep the stress down. Slow thought processes, inability to deal with extremes, damaged perceptual abilities and sensitivity to light can all be especially stressful while traveling. With stress and the increased LBD symptoms it can cause, travel becomes difficult if not impossible—and definitely no fun for anyone. On the other hand, the more comfortable the PwLBD is with the surroundings, the fewer problems there will be.

If you fly, buy travel insurance and be prepared to use it. If the PwLBD starts out feeling paranoid or frightened when getting on the plane, it isn't going to get better. Get off. DO NOT travel unless both of you feel well. It will almost assuredly make the disorder worse—and it may not bounce back. Stay home and "de-stress." Then try again.

Choose familiarity. Taking trips in a familiar vehicle to known places will be easiest. Adding anything strange increases stress. Thus, a trip made many times in the family car to see friends will be much easier than a trip on public transportation to a new destination. Adding unknown people, such as a tour group, increases the likelihood of stress. A person who is used to flying will be able to do so comfortably longer than a person who isn't.

Build in familiarity by taking along a well-liked blanket, favorite photos, and other such items to provide a feeling of home. Keep a regular routine. Even when the trip is in a less familiar mode of travel or to a less well known destination, these will help to decrease stress.

Avoid extremes—avoid anything too hot, too cold, too many people, too many noises, too excited, too tired, too anything. Follow the old adage, "Keep it simple." The fewer extremes, the less external confusion, the calmer the PwLBD can be. For instance, avoid a "five cities in ten days" type of trip and choose flights without stopovers whenever possible.

Is it real or is it a delusion? In an effort to make sense of confusion, the PwLBD may develop frightening delusions, which can feel absolutely true and be hard to correct. Hopefully, people with early LBD can give drivers and care partners the benefit of the doubt, even when sure that what they believe is right.

Jim and Annie were traveling in an area of rolling hills but Annie "saw" valleys and cliffs and believed Jim was driving much too close to the edge. In Chapter 12, Clark sincerely believed his wife was driving in the wrong direction, away from instead of towards home. In both cases, time made the difference. The terrain leveled out and Annie felt safe again. Clark and his wife made it home and Clark realized that he had been turned around.

Travel during optimal times. Take advantage of the times of day when the PwLBD is likely to be most functional. This is when to schedule outings, or to schedule the bulk of the traveling during longer trips. Scenery flashing by the windows of a fast moving car can be confusing and scary for a person with slow thought processing. If this fits, consider traveling at night, when there is less to see and when the PwLBD can sleep while the care partner drives.

Make it short. Shorter, closer to home outings may be more enjoyable than longer trips. Work as a team to plan for times when you both will enjoy traveling. On longer trips, go in short increments, with more time for resting up and adjusting between legs. Everything takes longer now. Without these built-in spaces, the PwLBD will feel rushed—and stressed.

Exercise. Traveling can be very confining and no one may get much exercise. Make a point of stopping often to walk around when traveling by auto. If going by air, spend time in the airport walking in the less populated areas or even outside. This will help to refresh you both and avoid stress. If mobility is already a problem, find a way to exercise in some way, even if it is no more than swinging arms around. Your bodies need that change from all the sitting that travel entails.

Look for the positives. With all the planning and effort, don't forget to enjoy your trip. Enjoy the beautiful scenery, the people, the food and each other. If that isn't possible, don't go!

Chapter 49

To Drive or Not to Drive

One of the hardest decisions a PwLB must make is when to stop driving. It may be more traumatic than asking someone else to handle financial decisions or even transitioning into assisted living. Getting a driver's license is a rite of passage into adulthood. Losing it can make a person feel less an adult.

The truth is that deciding to stop driving because it has become unsafe is very much an adult decision. Making that decision personally allows the PwLBD to feel more in control than if someone else must step in and take away the keys.

It used to be that a doctor who diagnosed a person with even mild dementia was required to notify the state Department of Motor Vehicles. In most cases, the state would then revoke that person's driver's license. This has changed as of 2010, when the American Academy of Neurology decided that a diagnosis of mild dementia did not necessarily mean that a person's driving ability would be impaired enough to be unsafe. They now recommend that in such cases, driving be evaluated every six months.

However, many people are never diagnosed with MCI even when they have the symptoms. Doctors hesitate to do so without a battery of tests to support their diagnosis. Since treatment is likely to be the same with or without the diagnosis, doctors tend not to push the tests unless there is a clear reason.

Understanding cause and effect. The decision about when to stop driving is usually something that a Lewy team must make.

The discussion about this should occur early in the journey, before the ability to understand cause and effect is gone. After that, the reasons for stopping will be too unclear to overcome the immediate advantages. Understanding cause and effect is an executive skill that the disorder can begin to erode early in the disease process.

Don't wait until others are concerned. Don't even wait for a LBD diagnosis to have this conversation. It is a discussion every Lewy team needs to have as soon as they know there is a risk of dementia in their future. Early on, both of you can be more objective and the discussion will be less traumatic. At this time, it will be easier to agree upon some red flags, some signs that driving has become unsafe. Agree also to review these red flags regularly. Finally, discuss what you will do when you begin to see these red flags.

When is it unsafe to drive?

The following questions provide some suggested red flags.

Does the PwLB:

- Avoid driving with grandchildren in the car?
- Drive fewer miles than he used to?
- Avoid driving at night, or in the rain, or in busy traffic, or in other situations that feel less safe?
- Get mad at other drivers easily, and do things like honk the horn, gesture or drive close to them?

Has the PwLB:

- Been the driver in an auto accident in the last three years?

- Received a ticket for a traffic violation like speeding or running a red light in the last three years?

Both team members should answer these questions. Any "yes" answers mean that driving may have become unsafe. The more yes answers, the more unsafe it probably is.[119]

Harold still believes that his driving is safe, but I don't. He used to be a very good driver but he is getting more careless and he gets much more impatient with other drivers. Sometimes he blames them for mistakes that he makes. -- Betty

Harold is a classic example of how people who desperately want to continue driving are seldom the best judges of their own ability. They tend to overlook serious issues as mistakes anyone can make once in a while, instead of the scary events that their passengers experience. Thus, Betty's red flag answers are probably the most correct.

If Parkinson's is involved, there could also be physical problems. A person needs to have adequate muscle control in legs, arms and neck to drive well. These abilities tend to decrease with stress, causing a person who may usually drive well to do poorly during a crisis—a time when safe driving is most needed.

Stopping driving. Although the PwLB may have agreed that when certain red flags appeared his driving should stop, it will seldom be an easy decision. However, its definitely worth the effort.

When I told Ted that I felt uncomfortable with him driving, he hit the roof. "I'm fine. I haven't run any stop signs have I?" he shouted. I almost lost my cool and yelled back. But instead,

I said, "Well, Dani and Joe asked me if you were safe to ride with." Dani and Joe are our daughter's kids. They are ten and twelve. "What?" he said. "Yes," I told him. "They have been worried too." He walked off but about a week later, he told me he didn't think he'd drive with anyone else in the car anymore. That's when I told him he was just as precious to me as the grandkids. He grinned and hasn't driven since. Of course, I made sure he "lost" his keys so he wouldn't be tempted or forget. --Jean

Mentioning grandchildren as Jean did will often get a PwLB's attention when a spouse's concern won't. Deciding to choose safety and the comfort of others over one's own needs is a very adult decision. It is another way to give the PwLB a feeling of being in control even when the choice itself is limiting. "Yes, Lewy is messing with my ability to drive, but I made the decision to quit. No one else made it for me."

Once the decision has been made to quit, make it happen right away. Like a bandage peeled slowly from a hairy arm, the longer the decision to quit is put off, the more painful it gets. Go the whole route. Get rid of the car keys. Allow the license to lapse. Do it now. Then there won't be that temptation to drive just one more time—and one more….

Teams often choose to put off this difficult decision until something happens and someone other than the caregiver can be the "bad guy" who insists that the PwLB's driving must end. Since no one can know if the precipitating event will be a mild fender-bender or a more serious accident, this isn't a very safe choice.

The part about making someone other than the caregiver the "bad guy" may be a good idea however.

I knew that if I did anything to keep Harold from driving, he would be very angry with me and so at his next doctor's appointment, I made it a point to talk privately to her about my concerns. She asked him if he was still driving. When he said he was, she warned him of the legal consequences of getting into an accident with a LBD diagnosis. Then she suggested that he either quit or get a driving evaluation. He chose to quit but he was really mad at the doctor. -- Betty

If the PwLB is not driving safely but is unwilling to stop, consider doing as Betty did and ask the doctor to step in. Then the PwLB can be mad at the doctor and not the care partner.

In a situation like this, respond to the PwLBD's feelings, and not to the relief you might feel. That is, commiserate about how awful it is to lose one's driving privileges. Do not talk about their driving being unsafe. That makes you the bad guy again.

LBD may have damaged a person's ability to comprehend cause and effect while leaving the immediate rewards of driving quite clear. "Safe driving" will have little meaning and a decision to quit will seem irrational. The person will likely be less willing or cooperative, especially if the issue hasn't ever been discussed previously.

While these earlier discussions about red flags may not be remembered when the time comes to act upon them, rest assured that they were not wasted. They are still there somewhere deep in the PwLB's subconscious and will truly make the final decision easier to accept.

Alternatives to Driving

During that early discussion about when to give up one's drivers license, talk about alternative transportation. Remember, the title of this section is "Getting On With Life." Shopping, visiting with friends and all other normal activities still go on. There simply needs to be a safer way to get there.

Often the solution is that the care partner can take over most of the driving. Most communities have handicap busses that can be scheduled for doctor's visits and other events. Some volunteer organizations offer driving services for people who can't drive. Talk to the local senior center staff. They will likely know who to contact. Having this information available when the time comes to go from driving to being a passenger will make that transition easier. Such transportation options to places like adult day care can also instill feelings of independence for the PwLBD while providing the care partner with some valuable personal time.

Chapter 50

Staying Active

Physical pastimes such as dancing, golf, tennis, or bowling gets the PwLB out with other people. With a change of focus from perfection to simply enjoyment, such pursuits enable the PwLB to continue to be active well into the LB journey. Review Chapter 29 for a list of ideas for continuing to be physically and socially functional. Here are some more suggestions for staying interested in life.

Creative activities. Encourage the PwLBD to continue to write or paint or do anything creative that they've always done. This is a wonderful way to express emotions while using a different part of the brain than that used for thinking.

> *I've been a writer all my life. For years, I wrote in long hand. I felt that it stirred my creative juices. When my writing became hard to read, I started typing. Lately, that became difficult. Now I dictate my stories and my dear wife transcribes them for me. It's become something we enjoy doing together. — Lester*

Lester and his wife aren't letting his disorder stop them. They continue to adapt.

> *Dad used to be a finish carpenter. He made all of my kitchen cabinets. But it got to where he wasn't safe with his tools anymore. I was afraid he was going to cut off a finger. We talked him into selling the power tools. Now I use a hand saw*

to cut boards for shelves and then he hand sands them. All of our friends are getting new shelves! — Patrick

Patrick's issue was safety. He had to step in and find a way for his dad to continue working with wood. His solution accomplished that and provided some quality father-son time as well.

Social activities. LBD may eventually make social activities less appealing because being around many people at a time is stressful. But don't give up. Arrange for visits with only one or two friends or family members at a time. It's worth the effort. Choose people who understand the PwLB's need for a calmer event. As with physical activities, goals must change. Once large crowds and loud events may have been fun and exciting. This will no longer be the case. A small intimate gathering, preferably at home will be much more enjoyable.

Chores and home projects. Gardening can be very invigorating. Use a raised platform if necessary. A project may not be so easy if it involves moving parts, but there are solutions.

My husband was the neighborhood fix-it man. Whenever anything went wrong with an appliance, the neighbors would call Andy. He could usually fix it. Now, his hands are too shaky to be able to do any of that, but he still likes to mess around with broken stuff like old clocks. — Rosalie

Andy stayed active by choosing something safe to work on. In addition, his focus changed from fixing to tinkering—from *finishing* a project to *having* a project. Staying busy and interested is what's important, not the end result.

Household chores offer many chances to stay active and be useful at the same time. Setting the table, clearing it, doing laundry and folding clothes are the ones that come to mind first.

Enjoy Life

Dealing with a Lewy body disorder is never easy. However, doing everything possible to help the Lewy team stay healthy, decrease stress and enjoy life will make it an easier, more enjoyable journey for everyone.

Section Ten:

Especially For the Care Partner

First you are a companion, then an occasional helper, and then without you really realizing what has happened, you may find yourself a full time caregiver. This section includes suggestions that can make your job easier.

Many things change, things that you may not expect. Rules change and the PwLBD's character may even change. The care partner's job also changes to include much that the PwLBD used to be able to do. But to survive, a care partner must take the time and effort for self care. This is not selfish—it is of prime importance to the PwLB. If the care partner becomes ill—or dies—who will be there for him.

Chapter 51

Rule Changes

LBD is a type of dementia where thinking errors, hallucinations and delusions can start early, well before obvious memory issues. This changes the rules.

Where reasoning and honesty were the basis of a good relationship, these may now cause dissention and stress. A PwLBD may angrily reject explanations in favor of his own erroneous conclusions. Impulsiveness and the inability to consider waiting for delayed gratification may leave him deaf to the voice of reason. He truly believes he has better cognitive powers than he does and demands to do things he can no longer do—like driving.

The Therapeutic Fib

In situations like these, care partners learn to use the "therapeutic fib" to maintain calmness and gain cooperation. Think of it as entering their reality. When you played make belief as a child, was that lying? No, it was your "reality" for that moment. This is much the same. The goal is to reduce the PwLB's stress—and in doing so, reduce your own.

> *I've never lied to Fred and I don't want to start now. But when I tell him that what he sees isn't really there, he gets agitated. — Katie*

Many couples have had a relationship like Katie's, built on honesty, reason and trust. LBD changes the rules. When the ability to reason is gone, honesty can become distressing instead of helpful. A PwLBD loses the ability to evaluate, consider the costs, or understand the problems involved. His world is concrete, black and white, yes and no. And so you must decide what to say, not by how true it is, but by how it will affect the PwLB. Trust remains, for any "lies" you tell will be in support of your loved one. The goal is always to decrease his stress—and your own.

> *Therapeutic fib:* The practice of entering the PwLBD's reality to present an issue in a way that will decrease stress and/or support good care. When used in this way, it should be considered a therapeutic intervention rather than dishonesty.

As the disorder changes, so do the rules.

Earl used to recognize that his hallucinations were false. Now he doesn't. He gets upset when he sees animals all over in our living room. I just open the door, shoo them all out and then tell him, 'OK, they're all gone now.' — *Julie*

Earl's inability to tell reality from fantasy is a sign that he is losing his ability to reason. Where once Julie may have been able to explain, now she is wasting your breath—and her patience. For Earl, what he sees is real. Period.

Sometimes you can avoid the truth or shade it a little. That's what Julie did. She didn't say, "Yes, there are animals in our living room," but in an implied lie, she joined in Earl's reality enough to get rid of his hallucinatory animals. See Chapter 11 for more about how to deal with hallucinations.

When I'm on the phone to anyone male, Richard accuses me of making plans to meet later and cheat on him. I've gotten so I just tell him it was my son. — Kendall

What Richard feels and believes is real to him. It would do no good for Kendall to deny that she was being unfaithful. In Dan's mind, her pleas of denial are lies—further evidence of unfaithfulness. See Chapter 12 for more about delusions. Kendall avoids the stress of an irrational confrontation by assigning her calls to an acceptable male, her son.

Shirley resists going to the doctor and so I tell her we are going out for an ice-cream treat. On the way, I stop at the doctor's, "just for a minute, to pick something up." Shirley doesn't like being left alone in the car and so it's easy to get her into the doctor's office. The nurse hustles us right into an exam room and the doctor shows up as soon as he can, saying, "While you were here, I just thought I'd come visit with you for a few minutes." It works like a charm!" — Clarence

Shirley can't make the connection between going to the doctor's office and her health. She only knows that she doesn't like going there.

Aaron resisted going to day care until I told him they needed him to work as a volunteer. The day care center was very helpful and knew just how to put him to work. I guess they get that a lot! — Jeanette

Aaron isn't able to understand that he needs to be supervised all the time or that his wife needs a break. Aaron simply knows he'd rather stay home. The daycare staff entered his reality and gave him a "job" that allowed him to feel useful and wanted.

When honesty can lead to distress for both caregiver and loved one, it stops being helpful. Was it harmful for Clarence to tell Shirley they were going out for ice cream and then sneak in a stop at the doctor's? Does it really matter if Aaron thinks that he is a volunteer at the day care center if it gets him there and helps him to feel useful? The answer to such questions is always "no, it doesn't matter and it isn't harmful *as long as it benefits the patient.*" This includes keeping the caregiver healthy and stress-free.

Care partners soon learn to develop a sense of humor and play along. With thinking errors in the picture, a PwLBD is beyond where honesty or dishonesty has any meaning. Whatever works, whatever is the least stressful, whatever gets the job done; that is what is right.

Bribery

When used with children, bribery is seldom a good solution. Mom tells Johnny that if he will stop crying, she'll give him a cookie. The immediate result is positive: he stops crying. However, when he wants another cookie, he's likely to start crying again. Therefore, the long term results are negative. That's because children can learn and use what they've learned for future experiences.

As dementia advances and learning becomes more difficult, this changes. The short term results are the only ones that count. Unlike when bribery is used with children, it is not a learning experience. It is simply a means to an end. Often it is a distraction. Sometimes it can be the way to get a loved one to do something they are resisting, as Clarence did to get his wife to go to the doctor. Don't be afraid to use it generously. Bribery works and has little or no negative backlash.

Punishment and discipline

Parents may use punishment to teach their children correct behavior. Children learn to avoid behaviors that will result in an unpleasant parental response. When "punished" with yelling or other ways to show disapproval, the PwLBD is likely to feel confused and hurt but won't have learned not to do the behavior again. With a fading understanding of cause and effect, the reason for the punishment gets lost and even if the PwLBD did understand, being able to remember not do the same behavior again is doubtful. In addition, yelling will be usually perceived as an attack, leading to increased agitation and acting-out.

This also includes discipline that is based on cause and effect.

> *I told Joe that he couldn't have his keys because he didn't drive safely anymore. He became very angry and said I just wanted to be mean. — Alice*

Joe comprehends only that he feels deprived and hurt. He probably can no longer understand the reasons why Alice thinks his driving is poor. Nor can he understand what his supposedly poor driving has to do with Alice withholding his keys. Unlike bribery, using punishment and teaching-oriented discipline with someone who can no longer reason not only doesn't work, it is counter-productive. Find another way to meet the need. For instance, Alice may have to "lose" the keys or even sell the car.

Decisions

The way families make decisions will often change, with the care partner taking more and more responsibility. Usually, this happens gradually but sometimes the time comes surprisingly early. Some decisions, like what to wear or eat will become too frustrating. Others, such as managing finances, medical and legal affairs will become unsafe.

When must the transition happen? When it becomes stressful or unsafe for the PwLBD to make the decisions, it is time for the care partner to take over. This can be a fairly painless transition if the team has done their homework and are prepared with the appropriate legal permissions. Without these legalities, it may take several disasters and many months to transfer the responsibility to the care partner. Chapter 17 in this book and Chapter 13 in the *Guide* provide the information you need to start this process.

Who makes the decisions when a parent can't? This may be a clear choice when the spouse or an only child is the caregiver. When adult children are involved, it can become murky. Just as they squabbled as young children about who did or didn't do the chores or got the best seat in the car, adult children may differ over how to care for their parents. Here are some tips about how siblings can share caregiving responsibilities:

- *Be aware.* Parents may fear losing independence so much that they don't ask for help. Discuss this with the family, preferably before the need arises.
- *Plan ahead.* Research the types of service, interventions or care options you may need. Talk with siblings about who

can do what. Divide up tasks and give everyone a chance to share their ideas. Discuss who can provide physical caregiving, who can provide funds for other needs, etc.

- *Be flexible.* Needs can change and responsibilities differ. Rather than insisting on an equal sharing of responsibilities, consider a division of labor that takes into account each sibling's interests, skills and availability.
- *Ask for help.* If you are the primary caregiver and it is becoming too much, speak up. Be specific about what would help. If a sibling can't help physically, can they pay for someone else to help, for instance?
- *Keep in touch.* If you are a long-distance sibling, check in frequently. Don't wait for the caregiving sibling to ask for help. Offer it often. Money is often the easiest but emotional support will often be equally as welcome.

Go to Caregiverstress.com[120] for a downloadable pamphlet on this subject.

At the doctor's office. In the past, the PwLB may have been in charge of making personal decisions about medical care. However, the time will come when the doctor needs to know more than the PwLBD can share. The care partner must step up and become a larger part of the treatment team.

> *Bob's doctor wants to just continue his meds but I think some of those drugs may be making Bob's delusions worse. I would like to discuss this with the doctor but hate to do it with Bob sitting there listening. I think it would just make him feel worse. – Joyce*

Talking about things such as delusions in front of the PwLBD is usually not productive and can be painful or even disastrous.

However, it is information the doctor needs to know. A Lewy-savvy doctor will solve this problem by making a time with just the care partner a part of every visit. When the doctor doesn't initiate this separate time for the care partner:

- *Ask for it when you make the appointment.* The time can be before or after a regular visit or totally different.
- *Use email or texting.* Arrange to email or text information you want known to the doctor prior to the visit.
- *Use the telephone.* Schedule a telephone conversation with the doctor for a time when you can talk privately.

Any time the care partner is sharing information about the PwLBD it should be accurate and specific. Use a journal to record events, with dates and times. Take it to all appointments and use it for reference when emailing, texting or telephoning.

> *Reminder:* All medical personnel must have legal permission, usually a medical Power of Attorney, before they can discuss their patient's medical care with anyone else, including a spouse or care partner.

Chapter 52

Character Changes

Like everything else about LBD, character changes are individual. No one's journey will be the same. In an extreme situation, the PwLBD can change from an independent, caring, polite person into a very dependent, selfish person with few inhibitions. Your experience may be milder, but do expect a certain amount of change. It can happen even during the early stages of the disorder before there are many obvious mental changes.

Think of the average two-year-old child. Children that age don't want Mommy out of their sight. They are quite stubborn about wanting their own way. They don't understand the concept of sharing or empathy—and they have few inhibitions. This is what dementia does to a person. It pulls them back into that space.

There are differences. Most importantly, the PwLBD is not a child and doesn't respond well when treated like one. He is also much stronger. Where you can pick a child up and move him out of harm's way, you can't do that with a 100-200 pound adult.

A two-year-old can learn. For the PwLBD, learning becomes more difficult, and is usually only possible with strong motivation and intense effort. Both of these attributes require an understanding of the need for change and that is gone too. Therefore, the care partner is the one who must adjust.

Acting-Out Behaviors

Unlike people with Alzheimer's, PwLBD often start acting out early in their journey. Hallucinations or delusions or even Active Dreams may initiate irrational responses such as anger or fear. As thinking becomes garbled and language skills decrease, communication abilities spiral downward. High stress levels increase the intensity of LBD symptoms and further decrease one's ability to communicate. Frustration adds to the intensity of the feelings and increases the behaviors.

Before using drugs to manage this behavior, try some other methods:

Check for physical influences. Injuries, fever, urinary tract or pulmonary infections, pressure ulcers (bed sores), and constipation can cause behavioral problems to suddenly grow worse.

Review current medication. Check both prescription and over-the-counter drugs. Certain sleep aids, strong pain medications, bladder control medications, and drugs used to treat LBD-related movement symptoms can cause confusion, agitation, hallucinations, and delusions. Similarly, some anti-anxiety medicines can actually increase anxiety in people with LBD.

> A normal dose of many behavior management drugs can be unsafe with Lewy body disorders. Actually, researchers are finding these drugs dangerous for the elderly in general.[121] It is easier to prevent unwanted behaviors than it is to manage them once they occur.

Change the care partner's behavior. To change a PwLBD's behavior, you must change your own behavior first—or perhaps it is better to say that you must change your attitude.

> *Once I understood that LBD was the culprit, my compassion and nurturing kicked in. Dan's reaction to my loving interactions, no matter what buttons he pushes, have really turned him around. I credit my change of attitude for making him so much easier to live with.* — *Janet*

Therapists talk about behavior modification. Be aware that it is the care partner's behavior that must be modified. The PwLBD can no longer change but his perceptions have increased. When you learn to become calmer and less confrontational, he will reflect this. Offering comfort and respect is also helpful.

> *If Dan is comfortable, he is peaceful and happy. If I respond in a way that makes him uncomfortable, it causes him agitation. I am still working on my behavior modification because every new thing he throws at me is a new thing to have to deal with. At first I may respond negatively but when I stop and think about what he is trying to communicate, then I can relax, apologize and get over it. He is not going to change for the better, so I might as well accept the changes that are occurring and deal with it in my own mind and with love.* — *Janet*

Janet recognized that Dan's behavior was often stress-related communication. You can find non-drug techniques suggested in Sections Three and Four to identify and change the conditions triggering the stress. Here are some reminders:

Change the triggering condition. Remove the trigger and the behavior will decrease and possibly stop.

> *Every time a certain aide entered Ted's room, he became violent. When he called her by the name of his first wife, I figured out that the poor innocent aide was bringing back memories of a painful divorce. I requested a different aide. That solved the problem. — Jean*

Jean knew it would be no good to try to explain to Ted that the aide wasn't his first wife. LBD had taken away his ability to reason. Luckily, the staff understood and was willing to try this before resorting to behavior management medications.

Speak to the intent, not the behavior. Once you know what the PwLBD is trying to say, it becomes easier to respond in ways that decrease rather than increase anxiety.

Consider temporary drugs. Sometimes drugs may be needed to quickly alter the PwLBD's behavior. Once the tension decreases, non-drug intervention will likely be more successful. It may take the physician time to find the right drug and dosage. Be aware that as LBD progresses, this will change. Using drugs with LBD is always a trial and error affair.

Stay safe. If you have done everything possible and still feel unsafe, call for help. This may mean calling a relative or friend, or more likely, it will mean calling 911. If so, expect your loved one to be transported to a hospital emergency room. Be prepared with the LBDA wallet card, and any other information you need. (See ER List in the Resource Section, under Drug Information and Forms.)

Dependence

As LBD progresses, your loved one will become much more dependent. This may happen well before he loses the ability to do things for himself. He may seem afraid to let you out of his sight. Caregivers call this "shadowing."

> *For about 18 months, I felt as though Ted and I were attached at the hip. He followed me everywhere. He hated it when I went into the bathroom and closed the door. I finally just left it open. It wasn't worth the battle. But then he changed, and he seemed happy to simply sit in his chair and watch TV.* — *Jean*

As Ted's sense of the world narrowed, Jean was his point of orientation. He needed to know where she was to know where he was.

Cycles

Caregivers report that things seem to go in cycles with LBD. Whatever the PwLBD is doing now, caregivers report that it can change at any time. For a while—a day, a week or longer—a PwLBD may be very dependent, as Ted was. Dependence will always be an issue, but the extreme dependence may disappear, to be replaced with something else. The PwLBD may have a period of being very delusional, may want to eat all the time or have sleeping issues that make him stay awake at night and want to sleep all day. Knowing about cycles may help you deal with any behavior you find more difficult than most. Keep in mind that "this too shall end."

Stubbornness

This goes along with the loss of thinking abilities. "What I know is what I know and what I want is what I want," is the mantra of the person with dementia. He can't be reasoned with, so don't try. The therapeutic fib and bribes comes into effect here. Just as a child can be enticed or distracted with a favorite food or toy, so can PwLBD. Join their reality, distract, bribe and rephrase.

Impulsiveness and Lack of Inhibitions

Children learn to control bodily functions, monitor what they say and use a variety of safety precautions. LBD takes these inhibitions away and leaves the PwLBD feeling free to impulsively do things such as pass gas in public, swear at the minister or dash out into the street without a bit of care.

The first is simply embarrassing. Just smile and shrug if anyone looks at you in askance. Susan Scarff designed what she called her "Yikes" card[122] to hand out in embarrassing situations. This computer generated business-sized card reads, "My husband has a brain disorder. Thank you for your patience." This might also help you deal with something more serious such as soothing an affronted minister.

Impulsivity can also show up in a sort of incontinence. Men may start urinating anywhere, even before they are actually incontinent. However, the solutions are the same as for regular incontinence—scheduled bathroom trips, signs for where the bathroom is, and diapers if necessary—and a smile, a shrug and a "Yikes card" when it happens in public.

Lack of inhibitions and impulsiveness can result in serious safety issues. Chapter 44 has some suggestions for safety-proofing your home. You can find articles with more ideas in the Resource Section under Home Safety. However, no matter how much you plan, something else will come up. Be prepared. Innovation is the name of the game!

Obsessive Compulsive Disorder (OCD)

This is different from impulsiveness, which is doing something without thinking about it ahead of time. OCD is the compulsive need to obsess upon a certain behavior and do it repeatedly, usually in response to hidden anxiety.[123] The behavior could be something as simple as checking and rechecking to see if a door is locked or a towel is folded correctly. Gambling, shopping, eating or sexual activity are common forms. Women are more likely to overeat and shop; men are more likely to gamble and be obsessed with sex.

Identify and reduce the anxiety. While not specifically a Lewy body-related symptom, OCD is a common response to the anxiety that can accompany any degenerative disorder. It is especially common for those with impaired thinking abilities. Identify the reason for the anxiety and reduce or change it. This may defuse the OCD. To prevent a buildup of anxiety, incorporate stress management tools and use them regularly. Since the PwLBD responds not only to their own stresses but mirrors the care partner's as well, this is a partnership activity. Both need to keep stress levels low.

Medication. OCD can be a side effect of certain medications. Parkinson's drugs, particularly Requip and Mirapex, but also Sinemet on a lesser scale, may sometimes cause an unhealthy level of gambling, shopping, eating or sexual activity.[124] When the drugs are stopped or decreased, the OCD behaviors may disappear. Times vary. The compulsive behavior may not show up for as long as a year after the start of a drug. Once the drugs have been adjusted, it can take from days to months for the behaviors to subside. When non-drug methods fail, some caregivers have reported success with the less dangerous antipsychotics such as Seroquel.

Build in limits. With each targeted behavior, limits will be different. If eating is the behavior, monitor the food in your home and limit what is available, with the focus on healthy choices. With gambling or shopping, limit the funds available. This may mean canceling or changing credit cards. Monitor your computer and use the parental controls to limit shopping and gambling sites.

Sexual Acting-Out

As cognitive abilities decrease, impulsivity and sensitivity to feelings increase. This is a combination that can increase libido and sexual needs. It may occur early on and continue for most of the LBD journey. Sexual arousal is a very primitive feeling and often one of the last to go. However, appropriate sex in our world requires the ability to make judgments, understand cause and effect and delay gratification. LBD usually affects these skills much earlier than it does one's reproductive system.

When impulsiveness replaces the above skills, feelings and perceived needs become all important while place, time and perhaps even person become moot. When confronted about the inappropriateness of sexual advances, the PwLBD will often show hurt feelings or anger, with little or no understanding of why they are being confronted. To make matters worse, the more demanding or dependent a PwLBD becomes, the harder it is for a care partner to respond sexually. Even so, most spousal caregivers say they try to accommodate their loved one. This may actually be good therapy.

If he can reach a climax, it relaxes him for several days and he requires less medication. Believe me this has nothing to do with me - I just lay there and snuggle! — Linda

There is scientific support for this spouse's statement. Sexually active couples in general tend to have less stress. It has to do with the feel-good hormones released on climax. Even if a care partner isn't in the mood, helping her husband to climax may make both of their lives easier for the next several days!

My husband of 48 years is mostly bedridden but he still wants sex now and then. It's the only time he expresses feelings. He holds me and tells me he loves me although I'm not sure he knows who I am. I just lay there and cuddle and think of it as a gift for my beloved husband who has lost so many other pleasures. — Annette

This couple is near the end of their LBD journey but other care partners, with more functional loved ones have similar stories. For some it is a way of bringing back better times. For others like the caregiver above, it is a gift.

We hold hands and touch a lot. That seems to decrease the amount of sex that he wants. — Louise

Along with the closeness, it may be that the PwLBD wants the assurance that his mate is still there for him.

Although it is not as common, women can also experience libido issues.

> *Our home health aide came to me and asked if she could bring in someone to satisfy my mom. She complains all the time about being "horny" and nothing seems to help. — Darlene*

As the need becomes more compulsive and demanding, the behavior is more distressing and more difficult to deal with, as shown in the next four examples:

> *My husband wants sex all the time. I have to stop whatever I'm doing and go in and just lay there and let him try to do his thing—which he usually can't. If I don't, he gets really mad and I'm afraid he'll hit me. This really makes me sad. He used to be such a gentle person. — Arla*

If like Arla, you have become concerned about your own safety and can't find an immediate solution, it is time to consider more help and possibly residential care.

> *I'm losing my friends. My husband, Brian, has started hitting on them, groping them and making suggestive remarks. I try to explain that it is the disorder, not him, but I guess they don't understand. — Fran*

Many caregivers report this sort of problem. Fran can start by explaining to her friends that it's not Brian but his disorder and give them permission to gently deflect his advances. If that isn't enough, she may have to do her socializing away from home to avoid further issues.

When I tell my husband I'm not in the mood, he says he's going to ask that other woman. It doesn't do any good to explain that there isn't any other woman—that it's really me all the time. What I'm really afraid of is that he'll start asking real other women! *— Karlene*

Karlene's husband is experiencing Capgras Syndrome, where he thinks his wife is really someone else who just looks like her. This is a common delusion with LBD. Karlene needs to make sure friends or paid caregivers who come into contact with her husband understand his behavior. Home health aides have usually dealt with this before and when forewarned, will seldom be upset.

Sexual acting-out can be a form of OCD, discussed earlier in this chapter. Check to see if medication is causing the problem.

My 80 year old dad was propositioning me and any woman he met. The doctor reviewed his meds and reduced his PD drugs. He's not nearly so compulsive about sex now. — Carol

Try distraction. As with any other OCD, logic isn't going to work.

I went out and bought a bunch of porn books and paraphernalia. That keeps him happy for hours at a time. — Nelda

Nelda's solution distracted her husband's attention from her to the paraphernalia. If that isn't a comfortable option, consider favorite foods, activities or videos.

Develop a routine and set limits. This requires that there is still an ability to delay gratification. If OCD started early, while cognitive abilities still function to some extent, this may work.

> *It doesn't work to tell him "not now" because he's lost the concept of time. He just asks again in five minutes. I finally told him "only on Tuesdays." Now he checks out the calendar —which he can no longer read--all day long. I just tell him this isn't Tuesday.* — Letty

"Not now" doesn't work and Letty's solution does work for the same reason: her husband doesn't understand the concept of time. He can't tell when "Tuesday" is. His attention span also is short, so he doesn't remember her previous responses.

Keep calm. Since a PwLBD mirrors feelings, respond to his demands in a quiet calm manner even when you want to shout. A smile, a pat on the arm and a "No, dear, but wouldn't it be fun to watch your favorite video?" will always work better than showing anger or frustration.

As with other OCDs, search out and reduce the hidden anxiety, lower stress and if necessary, ask the doctor about medication to decrease the behavior.

Chapter 53

Being an Advocate

The care partner's job includes advocating, or speaking up, for their loved one with the medical community and others. This will likely start while functioning is still good except during times of stress. Of course, most times when situations need explaining or questions need to be asked are stressful. Be prepared to step up and advocate.

Do your research. LBD is still a less than well-known disorder even in the medical community. Learn as much as you can about it. This applies especially to drugs that work and drugs that don't work with LBD in general and with your loved one specifically.

Keep a journal. Care partners may consider this one more job in an already over-filled day and skip it as unimportant. It isn't. An accurate and up-to-date daily journal will save time and anguish as you attempt to share information with others. It will give your words validity when Showtime makes it hard for others to believe you. It will help you to see where needs are that you might miss without this ongoing record. Your journal doesn't have to be lengthy. But it should record any difficult or unusual behaviors and reactions to medications.

Be alert. Being an advocate means being aware of what is going on so that you can speak up as needed. Weigh what others say against your knowledge of your loved one's situation.

Speak up. Almost always, medical personnel will know more about medical issues in general than most laymen. That's what you pay them for! However, through research and experience, many care partners become very knowledgeable about LB disorders and especially about their loved one's particular issues. Keep this in mind. Be brave enough to speak up and ask questions, and even make suggestions. The doctor may have reasons for the treatment that you haven't considered—or may change the treatment due to your concerns.

Use available resources. You aren't alone. You have the support of the LBDA via its wallet card and the articles on its site, and a caregiver's help line. Use your journal entries and the items in the Emergency Room List (Resources section, Drug Information and Forms) to give your requests validation.

Stay cool. The old adage "You can catch more flies with honey than vinegar" holds true. It also helps you to appear professional. This doesn't mean giving up. Just continue to repeat what you want without acting frustrated or angry. Being emotional decreases your effectiveness. You will be labeled hysterical and lose validity, making your job much harder.

Give credit where credit is due. Look for things to compliment and ways to give credit. When people hear honest positives, they are more open to hearing anything else you say and more willing to work towards a compromise.

Look for win-win ways. The goal is for your loved one to have the best treatment possible, not to get one-up on the doctors or other staff. This is more likely to happen when you work as a team, with all involved making an effort to do the best they can.

Chapter 54

Caregiver Care

Planning ahead is a good start towards self-care. However, it is much too easy to get caught up in the chaotic merry-go-round of caregiving and forget that you are responsible for two people not just one. You must take care of *yourself* as well as your loved one.

Caregiving is a team job. The PwLB is a member of the team and at first, the two of you will likely be enough. Together, you can get him up from the bed, down in his chair, dressed, fed and so on. Eventually, he will be able to help very little. Often what little help he provides makes more work, not less. That's when you desperately need to add another person to your team. It can be a family member, a friend, or a paid helper. But it must be someone you can count on regularly and someone your loved one can trust.

> ***Do not make the mistake of thinking that you can do caregiving alone.*** LBD care is never a one-person job and the need for more help will increase as the disorder advances.

The statistics show that many dementia caregivers die before their loved ones do. Usually, it is because they didn't put themselves first. They made sure their loved ones got to the doctor, but they "didn't have time to go" or "couldn't get away." They did everything they could to make life better for their loved one but neglected their own needs. They didn't use support groups, didn't take respite times, and ignored their health, their friends and their hobbies. When a care partner becomes ill and can't provide care anymore, the loved one is left without an anchor, without their small window of familiarity in an increasingly unfamiliar world.

Most of these caregivers would tell you they didn't have a choice. Their loved one needed everything they could give—and more; there just wasn't any time or energy left for anyone or anything else. They are wrong. It doesn't have to be that way.

The *Guide* has a large section on caregiver care. Begin using that information now, even before you really need to. Start by making routines and rituals that involve self-care.

When my mother was diagnosed with LBD, I realized that our family's journey might be a long one, and that it wouldn't be healthy to make LBD the total focus of our family life. To make my life during, and after, this journey better for me, I joined a support group. As a way of focusing on something other than my parents and their issues, my husband and I took on the project of establishing a large print library in the nursing home where my parents both lived. Later I became a volunteer with the LBDA and began managing its growing support group network. This gave me another outlet for my skills. I am convinced that joining a support group and carving out time to do meaningful and important volunteer work helped me 'come out the other side of my journey' stronger emotionally than I would have otherwise. — Ronnie Genser, LBDA 2009 Volunteer of the Year

Ronnie's suggestions are included in the following list of ways to keep maintain caregiver health:

Put yourself first. The caregiver's needs must take priority. Many care partners believe that their loved ones needs always come first. This is not true. A good care partner learns to be to put her own needs first and reframe "selfish" to "self care." Without this, the PwLB gets a defective, overworked, stressed out, often sick, caregiver. If you have so much to do that you aren't meeting your own needs, it is way past time to add another team member.

Join a support group. If your loved one has PD, start by attending the Parkinson's groups together. When dementia appears, look for a LBD caregiver support group. If there aren't any in the area, find a general dementia caregiver's group. These are often sponsored by the Alzheimer's Association. Don't forget the virtual groups listed on the LBDA website. These are especially valuable at three in the morning when your head is spinning with questions and concerns.

I don't know how caregivers manage without a support group. It is what keeps me going from month to month. I've made friends, learned about resources and most of all, had a chance to vent and share with people who are going through the same kinds of stuff I am. — Kim

Find an activity in which you can become emotionally invested. Not everyone can be so invested that they become Volunteer of the Year as Ronnie did, but do find an activity interesting enough that it will temporarily take your focus away from the day to day issues of caregiving. It doesn't have to be volunteer work, or even work, but it should be meaningful, as well as interesting and exciting. It doesn't even have to take much time, but it must be something that is important enough to you that you can focus on and think about It—instead of caregiving.

Have other interests. In addition to the above, maintain some less demanding interests outside of caregiving and set aside time for them. Choose something that you find relaxing or fun. It can be something as simple as reading a thriller or romance novel or something you've loved to do for years such as painting. It can be something you do alone, such as gardening. Or it can be something you do with others, such as playing cards. Getting your mind off caregiving even for short periods of time is a great stress reliever.

Include the PwLB in your planning. Early in the journey, you will likely make decisions as a team. Even though as time goes by, you will more often than not be the one who ultimately makes the decisions, don't stop the discussions. For your loved one, the feeling of being a part of the decision-making process will result in more willingness to follow through even when the memory of the discussion fades. For you, these discussions will decrease your feelings of being alone on this journey and make it easier to do what needs to be done without feeling so guilty.

Keep your *doctor's appointments.* Make regular doctor visits a habit. Set the appointments well ahead, put them on your calendar and make them priorities. Then, follow the doctor's orders. (That may be the hardest part!)

Make the time. Even if you aren't a full-time caregiver, you likely have a full life, with spouse, family and job. Whatever your situation, you need to make time for yourself. Start a routine of taking a few hours a week or even an occasional overnight away from caregiving and other responsibilities early in the LB journey. If this becomes an expected routine, it will not be so hard on either of you later. Make this a priority. It may mean asking for help. If you can't find time, then your team isn't functioning well. Do you need another team member? Is it time to ask the family for more help? Hire another caregiver? Add more hours for the caregiver you already have? Consider residential treatment?

Ask for help. Believe it or not, asking for help is an integral part of the caregiver's job. You can't do it all yourself. Delegate. Reach out to family and friends and let them know what you need. The most common need is for someone to come stay with your loved one for a while to give you some free time. This will seldom happen unless you ask. Others often don't see the need or don't know how to offer.

For most people, it isn't easy to ask for help. Even when someone offers it, the average person will deny the need. This is especially true when the offer is nebulous.

> *My friends would ask me how they could help and I'd tell them thanks for the offer but I'm doing fine. I wasn't, but I didn't know what to tell them. Then one day when I was*

doing some dishes that had piled up over a couple of bad days, I thought, "Gee, I'd sure like it if someone would come in and do these for me." I decided to make a wish list. I included things like doing the dishes, sitting with Earl for a while, vacuuming the floors, running errands, even bringing in a casserole. Now when anyone asks me how they can help, I just show them the list. It works! My friends like knowing what they can do and I get the help I need. – Lavita

Lavita's list makes it easy for her to respond to offers of help. She doesn't have to think of something right then. It is all laid out and her friends can choose what they'd like to do—or suggest something else.

I've found that my list often stimulates my friends to come up with their own ideas once they know I'm open to their help. A beautician friend offered to wash and cut my hair. Another friend offered to take Earl for a drive once a week. – Lavita

Asking for financial help may also be a part of the job. Distant relatives who can't help physically but they may be willing to help pay expenses—if they know the need. Think of this as offering them a way to be involved, rather than asking for a handout.

Another way a distant friend or family can help is to lend an ear. Caregiving can be isolating and it really helps to have someone who is willing to listen. They don't have to offer any solutions. Explain to them that just being able to talk to someone who will listen with no more than a supportive word now and then can be a great stress reliever.

Pay for help. Eventually, you will need more than the few hours of help that family and friends are usually able to provide. Plan for getting that help long before you need it physically. This is not a waste of money. It will pay for itself later. Your loved one will be better able to accept your absence when it is part of a known routine. Think of it as paying now for free time or paying later for stress-related illnesses. It truly is that serious.

Use your resources. There are many free or low cost resources for caregivers in most communities. Meals on Wheels provides meals to shut-ins and seniors in many areas. Dance classes are offered by many PD groups. Check with the Area Agency on Aging, Senior Centers, Alzheimer's and Parkinson's groups and any other similar organization. If these groups don't have services that can help, the staff will know who does.

Take regular respite "holidays." Set up a respite routine with someone your loved one trusts to take your place longer than just an hour now and then. It is best to make the time last at least overnight. It should also be something regular, something you can plan for. Depending on your finances, needs and wishes, these times away may be only a few hours a week or a couple of days a week, or more likely somewhere in between.

> *When I retired from my job to care for my sister, I knew even then how important respite was. Right from the first, we agreed that I would take off a couple of days a week. As my sister's health degenerated, I found that I didn't want to be away that long. I often shortened my respite to a single overnight or even just a few hours here and there but I never quit entirely. The time off made me a better caregiver. —* Helen Whitworth

As the situation at home changes, respite plans may also change. It will be tempting to give them up altogether at time. Shorten them if necessary, but don't quit. You need the "away time" to unwind and de-stress.

Have a caregiver backup plan. When building a respite routine, plan for emergencies as well. You may become ill, need surgery or be called away for some reason. Who will take your place? Knowing in advance that someone is available to stay with your loved one in these situations will decrease stress for both of you.

Get any remaining legal or financial papers completed. Having legal authority for the PwLB's care and finances will save multiple headaches. Don't put it off! (See Chapter 17 for specifics.)

Don't lose your sense of humor. Humor is a stress reliever. It makes everything a little bit easier.

Chapter 55

What If the Bottom Drops Out?

LBD fluctuates. That's expected. Fluctuating is one of its defining symptoms. Then there comes a day when the PwLB's functioning takes a long slide downward, with much more confusion, agitation, sleep problems and less mobility. (See the *Guide*, page 49.)

When this happens suddenly, not just the PwLBD but the whole team will be in crisis. Care partners won't be able to think clearly either. While they may know intellectually that people seldom gain back more than a fraction of the losses incurred during these sudden slides, it will be difficult to face such a quick degeneration. "Fluctuations happen and upturns follow downturns," or "With us, it will be different," worried care partners tell themselves, forgetting Lewy's relentlessly degenerative character.

Any number of situations can bring about these sudden downturns: illnesses as simple as a cold or as serious as kidney stones; a fall or a painful injury; ongoing problems like UTIs, dehydration or even a supposedly good thing like too much excitement over a happy event.

The cause may be nothing identifiable. A healthy, low stress lifestyle can extend cognition and make life much more enjoyable for a long time but does not necessarily extend life. When the reserves built up by careful living are gone, a PwLBD's mind and body degenerate very quickly. It is no one's fault. It is the nature of the disorder.

This is another turning point for which the Lewy team needs to prepare, earlier than later. It is easier to think that things will go gradually downhill, with expected fluctuations but nothing drastic. While they likely will, perhaps for years, the chances are that eventually, a slide will happen. What will you do then? How will you deal with these new, overwhelming problems that require so much energy, time and attention? Preparing for a downturn now does not mean that you expect or want one to happen. It means that you know it could happen and that by being prepared, you won't add to the problem by being so quite so stressed.

Know when to get help. These slides tend to sneak up on the team.

> *A couple of friends came in to sit with John while I ran some errands. When I returned, they both confronted me. "How do you do this 24/7?" they demanded. It was a wakeup call for me. I realized that I did need to get help. It was too much for one person to do alone anymore. — Pat Snyder[125]*

Pat had become so embroiled in just getting by day to day that she failed to see that her job has turned into more than she could safely handle. To avoid Pat's mistake, make a list that you check daily. If you answer yes to any of these questions, it is time to call for help:

- Has it been more than a week since the slide, with little or no recovery or worse, more decline?
- Am I are feeling overwhelmed by the physical requirements of caregiving?
- Am I getting so little sleep that my caregiving has suffered?

- Am I less patient or far too easy to anger?
- Do I feel that there aren't enough hours in the day for everything I need to do? Do I seldom take anytime just for me? Am I too tired to enjoy it when I do?
- Do a few hours of respite fail to rejuvenate me? Do I come back irritable and exhausted?

Know where to get help. Develop a list of places and people that may provide the help you will need. Call now, while not in crisis and find out about the services available. Sort them out by groups and grade them so that you will have a first and second choice when the time comes.

Respite care: You may already have friends or family coming to stay occasionally. After a slide, this will seldom be enough. You will need more than a few hours of time often clouded by worry that your helper won't know what to do if something goes wrong. Regular care with knowledgeable caregivers should start as soon as possible. If you choose respite care in a long term care facility instead of at-home help, the same issues apply as those used to find regular long term care. (See page 175 in the *Guide.*)

Reduce stress by keeping change at a minimum. If you plan to use home care, start it immediately for a few hours a week—enough to build a relationship with the helper. If you plan to use respite care, start visiting the facility with the your loved one. Go to lunch or dinner there. Even "take a vacation" together and visit overnight.

Equipment. The PwLB may suddenly need a wheelchair, a bathroom commode, a hospital bed or even a lift. Know where you can get these supplies. Physicians can write prescriptions so that Medicare will cover much of the cost. Find out now what the process is for this to happen. For example, can you call in a request or does the doctor need to see your loved one and evaluate the need?

Hospice. This may sound extreme, but it is also practical. Hospice offers the services and equipment you need to make your loved one comfortable and you less stressed.[126]

> *Walter suddenly got really bad. The doctor told us the end was likely near and so Walter went on Hospice in our own home. I got really depressed. I checked out funeral homes and looked at urns. Although Walter never totally recovered from his downturn, he did get so much better that after a few months he no longer qualified for hospice. He lived another two years, going back on hospice for the last six months. I still attend the grief groups. — Joan*

Hospice requires a doctor's documentation that death is likely within 6 months. Many people, including those with LBD, recover enough that they go off hospice and live for many months or even like Walter, for years longer. That's because hospice is designed to decrease stress and we all know what stress does to the Lewy team!

Change your view of hospice from something to bring into play when there's no more hope to seeing it as a practical use of available services. Using hospice is not an admission of failure or even an acceptance that the end is coming very soon. Instead, hospice can provide a multitude of help in a variety of ways, including nursing care, psychological support and more. Hospices vary in the services they provide. See the *Guide*, page 216.

Moving On

This book ends but life keeps moving on. Your Lewy team's journey will likely last many more years. Make it your primary job to keep those years as stress free and comfortable as possible. In that way, the team will have a more normal life, with less confusion and more clarity for your loved one and less work for you. So far, it isn't possible to stop the progression but you can definitely increase quality of life. That must be your goal.

In the meantime, check out our blog, Lewy Body Rollercoaster. There's a new entry every week, with current information, suggestions and ideas and new research about LBD.

Resources

Those using an e-reader connected to the internet can go to a site by clicking on its *italicized title*. This whole Resource list is online at *lbdtools.com/mcibook.html*. You can also type the provided web address (in parentheses) into your computer's address line and follow the directions.

Brain Donation Sites

Go to the web address shown, enter "brain donation" into the search box in the upper right hand corner and choose the first entry unless directed otherwise.

Brain Support Network. (brainsupportnetwork.org) Contact this group first. They provide complete, detailed brain donation arrangements tailored to the specific person and diagnosis, and support the entire way. robin.riddle@brainsupportnetwork.org, 650-814-0848.

Banner Sun Health Research Institute. (BannerHealth.com) Sun City, AZ. 623-832-6528 or 623-832-6511.

Boston University School of Medicine, (bu.edu/research) Alzheimer's Disease Center. Boston, MA. 888-458-2823.

Northwestern University, Chicago, IL (brain.northwestern.edu) Choose "Brain Endowment" in the Research & Clinical Trials sidebar. 312-926-1851.

University of California, San Francisco. (ucsf.edu) Click "ucsf" under the search box. San Francisco, CA. 415-476-1681.

Caregiver Information

American Parkinson Disease Association. (apdaparkinson.org/ information-referral-centers) Lists PD medical and research centers by state.

AssistGuide Information Services (AGIS) (agis.com) Excellent site with checklists, databases, information, and other caregiver support.

Caregiver Action Network. (caregiveraction.org). Their Caregiver Toolkit contains many guides such as Managing Medication or Financial Planning. 202-772-5050.

Disability.gov. (disability.gov) A comprehensive Federal website of disability-related government resources.

Eldercare Online. (ec-online.net) Provides state by state databases of government, county and local services available as well as other information. 631-224-7262.

Family Caregiver Alliance. (caregiver.org) One of the best caregiver sources on the internet. Find database for a multitude of local resources by state in the right hand panel (with map). 800-445-8106.

Health Finder.gov. (healthfinder.gov) Provides links to selected online publications, clearinghouses, databases, websites and support and self-help groups, as well as government agencies and nonprofit organizations for seniors and others.

National Association of Area Agencies on Aging. (n4a.org) Offers a variety of services to seniors. Most areas will have local offices. 202-872-8888.

NIH Senior Health. (nihseniorhealth.gov) National Institute of Health website provides aging-related health information for adults 60 and over.

Teepa Snow: Positive Approach to Brain Change. (teepasnow.com) A great source of ideas for dementia care, stress management and general caregiving.

Teepa Snow's Free YouTubes. (lbdtools.com/resources.html) A link to a list of these very helpful short videos. Find the longer versions for sale in the LBDtools.com store.

U.S. Administration on Aging. (aoa.gov) Site contains a wide array of information on older persons and services for the elderly. Several resource rooms focusing on such topics as Alzheimer's disease and caregiving are available. 202-619-0724.

USA.gov for Seniors. (USA.gov/Topics/Seniors.shtml) Website helps users access all government sites that provide services for senior citizens, including caregiver's resources, federal and state agencies for seniors, health, laws and regulations, housing and end-of-life issues. 800-FED-INFO or 800-333-4636.

Clinical Trials

Fox Trial Finder. (foxtrialfinder.michaeljfox.org) Online resource to help people find opportunities to participate in Parkinson's clinical trials.

NIH Clinical Research Trials and You. (nih.gov/health/clinicaltrials) Information about clinical trials, why they matter and how to participate. Find information about the basics of clinical trial participation; first hand experiences from actual clinical trial volunteers; explanations from researchers; and links on how to search for a trial or enroll in a research matching program.

US Information on Clinical Trials and Human Research Studies. (clinicaltrials.gov) A nationwide database allows you to search by name, medical condition, or your location.

Drug Information

Drug interaction checkers. Check for interactions between two or more drugs on any of the next four sites, All include prescription and OTC drugs, supplements, and some foods.

CVS. (cvs.com) Click on "Drug Information Center" for drug interaction checker, pill identifier and individualized medicine list.

Drugs.com. (drugs.com) Interaction checker lists all interactions for a single drug with severity as well as checking for interactions between an individualized list of drugs. By signing in, you can accumulate information from successive searches. Also offers a pill checker.

Health Line. (healthline.com) Click on "Drug Search" for interaction checker, pill identifier and drug comparison tools.

Walgreens. (walgreens.com) Click on "Pharmacy and Health" tab, then in the blue sidebar, scroll to "Health Center" and choose "Check Drug Interactions." Sign in to check interactions with your entire prescription history.

Anticholinergic drug lists. To access the following three sites, enter the *complete title* into a search engine.

The Revised Beers Criteria (Medication List). Revised by the American Geriatric Society in 2012, this extensive list shows drugs by use, and quality of evidence but not brand names.

The Anticholinergic Cognitive Burden Scale (PDF). Last updated in late 2011, this scale divides anticholinergic risk into three levels. A second scale divides the risks into Possible and Definite. Neither gives brand names or drug uses.

Anticholinergics and the Elderly-Detail document. Compiled in 2011 from several other sources, this scale shows brand names, drugs uses and levels of anticholinergic risk.

Drug Alert Information and Forms

Emergency Room List: (lbdtools.com/resources.html) A list of documents to take with you when you visit an ER or any other place where the staff may not be familiar with LBD.

Hospital Form. (lbdtools.com/resources.html) Download this form, fill it out and put it in your Emergency Room packet.

LBDA Medical Alert Wallet Card. (lbda.org/content/lbd-medical-alert-wallet-card) Carry this card with you everywhere.

Publications for Professionals. (lbda.org/content/publications-professionals) A list of articles and checklists designed especially for professionals. Good articles to copy and give to doctors and other medical staff.

Treating Psychosis in LBD. (lbda.org/go/ER) Download this and add it to your Emergency Room packet.

Why Do Many People with LBD Respond Poorly to Surgery?
(http://lbda.org/content/ask-expert-why-do-many-people-
lbd-respond-poorly-surgery) From LBDA's Ask the Expert. A
good article to copy and give to anesthesiologists and
surgeons when considering surgery.

Drug and Medical Assistance Programs

Drug Costs. (medicare.gov) Choose "Your Medicare Costs",
then "Save on drug costs" in the blue sidebar. Information
about public and private programs that offer discounted or
free medication, programs that provide assistance with other
health care costs, and Medicare health plans that include
prescription coverage.

Medicare.gov. (medicare.gov) The Official U.S. Government
Site for People with Medicare.

GovBenefits.gov. (govbenefits.gov) This official government
benefits website is a free, confidential tool that helps
individuals find government benefits they may be
eligible to receive.

Social Security Administration. (ssa.gov) The toll-free number
is live 7AM to 7PM EST, Monday to Friday. Recorded
information and services are available 24 hours a day. The
website provides a wealth of information and resources
including many databases and publications. 800-772-1213.

Together Rx Access. (togetherrxaccess.com) Several drug
companies have partnered together to provide a drug card
program that offers discounts on prescription drug purchases
for uninsured Americans. 800-444-4106.

Veterans Administration. (va.gov). Site provides information on VA benefits and services such as Aid & Attendance. 800-827-1000.

HelpRx.info. (http://www.helprx.info/discounts). Site offers card and coupons to print and take to your pharmacist to help with the cost. While *pharmacies are not required to honor discounts*, reviews show they usually do, at least in part. This site can be especially helpful for the person without insurance.

Home Safety

Assist Guide Information Services (AGIS) (agis.com/Eldercare-Basics).In the blue sidebar, choose "Staying at Home," then , "Improving your home." Includes several safety checklists. 866-511-9186.

Everyday Health.com (everydayhealth.com) Enter "home safety Alzheimer's" in the Search box in the upper right hand corner for several articles on home safety with dementia.

National Institute on Aging. (NIA) (nia.nih.gov/Alzheimers/) Choose "Publications," then enter "home safety" into the *Keyword box (not* the Search box in the upper right hand corner). Safety information applies to anyone with cognitive or movement disorders.

Legal Help

Caring Connection.org. (caring connection.org). Download free printable advance directive and instructions. 800-658-8898.

Five Wishes. (agingwithdignity.org) Choose a free online or buy a printed personalized booklet with advanced medical directive for $5. 888-5WISHES or 800-594-7437.

U.S. Living Will Registry. (uslwr.com/formslist.shtm) Advance directive forms by state. Offers a $5 registry program helpful if you travel a lot.

The National Academy of Elder Law Attorneys, Inc. (NAELA). (naela.org). Click on "About," " Consumer" and "Find a Lawyer." Lists elder care lawyers.

Long-Term Care and Placement

A Place for Mom. (aplaceformom.com) Senior care by state. Sign in to receive free personalized recommendations.

Assist Guide Information Services (AGIS) (agis.com) 866-511-9186. Choose the "Find Facilities and Services" tab, then enter "Assisted Living" and your location into the Local search box. Search for various types of LTC listed for each community and up to 50 miles away. No reviews.

Guide to Long Term Care for Veterans (va.gov) Enter "long term care guide" into the search box in the upper right hand corner. Information about long term care options, home and community based, and residential care.

Nursing Home Comparison. (medicare.gov/NHCompare) Detailed information about the past performance of every Medicare and Medicaid certified nursing home in the country.

National Organizations by Disorder

Parkinson's Disease

American Parkinson Disease Association. (apdaparkinson.org) Information and referral centers in many states. Lists PD health centers by state. 135 Parkinson Avenue, Staten Island, NY 10305. Email: apda@apdaparkinson.org . 718-981-8001 or 800-223-2732

Bachmann-Strauss Dystonia & Parkinson Foundation. (dystonia-parkinsons.org) Focus is on research and spreading awareness. Fred French Building 551 Fifth Avenue at 45th Street, Suite 520, New York, NY 10176.Email: info@bsdpf.org. 212-682-9900.

Davis Phinney Foundation. (davisphinneyfoundation.org) Partners with other organizations to provide information, tools and inspiration and fund research. 4676 Broadway, Boulder, CO 80304. Email:info@davisphinneyfoundation.org. 866-358-0285 or 303-733-3340.

Melvin Weinstein Parkinson's Foundation. (mwpf.org) Equipment and supplies for PD patients. Partnered with the PDF, via the Helen M. Lynch Direct Aid Fund. 757-496-7946.

Michael J. Fox Foundation for Parkinson's Research. (michaeljfox.org) Funds research. Grand Central Station, P.O. Box 4777, New York, NY 10163. 212-509-0995

National Parkinson Foundation. (parkinson.org) Research, education and outreach. 1501 N.W. 9th Avenue, Bob Hope

Road, Miami, FL 33136-1494. Email: contact@parkinson.org. 305-243-6666 or 800-327-4545

Parkinson Alliance. (parkinsonalliance.org) Fundraising for research. P.O. Box 308, Kingston, NJ 08528-0308. 609-688-0870 or 800-579-8440.

Parkinson's Action Network (PAN). (parkinsonsaction.org) Lobbyists for Parkinsons. 1025 Vermont Ave., NW, Suite 1120, Washington, DC 20005. Email: info@parkinsonsaction.org. 800-850-4726 or 202-638-4101.

Parkinson's Disease Foundation (PDF) (pdf.org) Research, education and public advocacy. 1359 Broadway, Suite 1509, New York, NY 10018. Email: info@pdf.org. 212-923-4700 or 800-457-6676.

Parkinson's Resource Organization. (parkinsonsresource.org) Support groups in CA. 74-478 Highway 111, No 102, Palm Desert, CA 92260. Email: info@parkinsonsresource.org. 760-773-5628 or 877-775-4111.

The Parkinson's Institute and Clinical Center. (thepi.org) Specializes in PD treatment and research. 675 Almanor Avenue, Sunnyvale, CA 94085. Email: info@thepi.org. 408-734-2800 or 800-655-2273.

Worldwide Education & Awareness for Movement Disorders (WE MOVE) (wemove.org) 5731 Mosholu Avenue, Bronx, NY 10024. Email: wemove@wemove.org. 347-843-6132

Lewy Body Dementia

Lewy Body Dementia Association (lbda.org) An excellent source of LBD Caregiver information and support. Many local support groups. Helpline: 800-LEWY SOS (539-9767). Office: 404-935-6444.

Lewy Body Society. (lewybody.org) A United Kingdom organization with the mission of raising awareness of LBD throughout Europe.

Lewy Body Foundation. (lewybodyfoundation.wordpress.com) An Australian group that proposes to fund research on LBD and Parkinson's disease.

LBDA Caregiver Forums (lbda.org/forum) These forums are not private. Anyone can read them. Join to post questions or comments.

Caring Spouses Yahoo Group (groups.yahoo.com) Enter "Caring Spouses" in the Search Groups box at the top of the page. A private group limited to spouses of LBD patients.

LBD Caregivers Yahoo group (groups.yahoo.com) Enter "LBD Caregivers" in the Search Groups box at the top of the page. A private group open to anyone interested in LBD caregiving, including spouses and professionals.

Facebook Lewy Body Dementia Support Group, (facebook.com) Enter "Lewy Body Dementia Support " in the Facebook search box. A closed group, easy to join. For anyone interested in LBD.

Alzheimer's Disease

Alzheimer's Association. (alz.org) Nationwide Local Chapters and Caregiver Support Groups. Helpline:800-272-3900.

Alzheimer's Foundation of America. (alzfdn.org) Social Worker Helpline: (Also available via Skype, live chat or email. 866-232-8484.

Alzheimer's Disease Education and Referral (ADEAR)
Center. (alzheimers.org) Sponsored by the National Institute
of Health, this site provides a current, comprehensive,
unbiased source of information about Alzheimer's disease.

Frontotemporal Disorders

The Association for Frontotemporal Degeneration.
(theaftd.org) Provides accurate information, compassion and
hope when lives are touched by any type of FTD. Helpline
email: info@theaftd.org. Helpline: 866-507-7222.

Early-Onset Dementia

Early LBD Virtual Support Group. (lbda.org/forum) A
private sub-forum on the LBDA.org website for those with
early LBD. In the Living with LBD section.

Early-Onset Caregiver's Support Group. (groups.yahoo.com)
Enter "Early Onset Caregiver" in the Search Groups box at
the top of the page to access group. A private online support
group for caregivers of people with early onset dementia of
any kind.

Memory People, Facebook group. .(facebook.com) Enter
"Memory People" in the search box. Started by Early Onset
AD patient Rick Phelps. A private place where patients with
early dementia and caregivers share experiences and concerns.

The Alzheimer Spouse (thealzheimerspouse.com) A private
group started for EOAD spouses. Also available to spouses of
people with other early onset dementias

Index

References

Find a digital copy of this list on the LBDtools website at www.lbdtools.com/links.html.

[1] **Savica R, et al.** (2013) Incidence of Dementia With Lewy Bodies and Parkinson Disease Dementia. JAMA Neurol. 2013; doi:10.1001/jamaneurol.2013.3579.

[2] **Span P.** (2012) A Form of Dementia That Is Often Misdiagnosed. New York Times, New Old Age, September 25, 2012. http://newoldage.blogs.nytimes.com/2012/09/25/a-form-of-dementia-that-is-often-misdiagnosed/

[3] **Lippa C, et al.** (2007) DLB and PDD boundary issues: Diagnosis, treatment, molecular pathology, and biomarkers. Neurology 2007;68;812-819. http://www.grg-bs.it/usr_files/eventi/journal_club/programma/dlb07.pdf

[4] **Hake, AM.** (2011) Dementia with Lewy bodies: Historical note and nomenclature. http://www.medmerits.com/index.php/article/dementia_with_lewy_bodies/P1

[5] **Barrett P. and Greenamyre JT.** (2014) Gene-environment Interactions in Parkinson's Disease. The Dana Foundation. http://www.dana.org/Publications/ReportOnProgress/Gene-environment_Interactions_in_Parkinson%E2%80%99s_Disease/

[6] **Tanner C.** (2011) Environmental Factors and Parkinson's: What Have We Learned? News & Review, Spring 2011, Parkinson's Disease Foundation. http://www.pdf.org/en/environment_parkinsons_tanner

[7] **Federal Register.** (2013) Secondary Service Connection for Diagnosable Illnesses Associated With Traumatic Brain Injury. Federal Register, Volume 78, Number 242 (Tuesday, December 17, 2013)Rules and Regulations, Pages 76196-76209. http://www.gpo.gov/fdsys/pkg/FR-2013-12-17/html/2013-29911.htm

[8] **National Cell Repository for Alzheimer's Disease.** (2013) 10 Things You Should Know about Lewy Body Dementias. Adapted from the LBDA for NCRAD Update,19, 4-2013. http://ncrad.iu.edu/Newsletters/PDFs/201304_NCRADUpdate.pdf

[9] **Grathwohl A, et al.** (2013) Mind the gut: secretion of alpha-synuclein by enteric neurons. Journal of Neurochemistry, 2013, 125, 487-490. http://onlinelibrary.wiley.com/doi/10.1111/jnc.12191/pdf

[10] **Ferman TJ, et al.** (2013) Non-amnestic mild cognitive impairment progresses to dementia with Lewy bodies. Neurology. 2013 Dec 3;81(23):2032-8. http://www.ncbi.nlm.nih.gov/pubmed/24212390

[11] **Miyamoto T, et al.** (2011) Idiopathic REM Sleep Behavior Disorder: Implications for the Pathogenesis of Lewy Body Diseases. Parkinsons Dis. 2011; 2011: 941268. http://www.ncbi.nlm.nih.gov/pmc/articles/PMC3096138/

[12] **National Institute of Neurological Disorders and Stroke.** (2012) Multiple System Atrophy Fact Sheet. http://www.ninds.nih.gov/disorders/msa/detail_msa.htm

[13] **Vya U and Franco R.** (2012) REM Behavior Disorder (RBD) as an Early Marker for Development of Neurodegenerative Diseases. BJMP 2012;5(1):a506. http://www.bjmp.org/content/rem-behavior-disorder-rbd-early-marker-development-neurodegenerative-diseases

[14] **Chiasson G.** (2002) Parkinsonian Syndromes. CME Case Study. The Canadian Journal of CME, July 2002. http://www.stacommunications.com/journals/pdfs/cme/julycme/e.pdf

[15] **NHS Choices.** (2011) Corticobasal degeneration. NHS, Health A-Z. Last reviewed 22/12/11. http://www.nhs.uk/Conditions/Corticobasal-degeneration/Pages/Introduction.aspx

[16] **NIH Publication No. 11-3897.** (2011) Progressive Supranuclear Palsy Fact Sheet, NINDS, May 2011. http://www.ninds.nih.gov/disorders/psp/detail_psp.htm#184703281

[17] **Lewy Body Dementia Association.** (2013) Common Forms of Dementia. http://www.lbda.org/node/8

[18] **University of California, San Francisco.** (2012) Frontotemporal Dementia, Overview. http://memory.ucsf.edu/ftd/overview

[19] **Alzheimer's Association.** (2014) 2014 Alzheimer's Disease. Facts and Figures. http://www.alz.org/downloads/Facts_Figures_2014.pdf

[20] **Lewy Body Dementia Association.** (2012) Genetic Variant Increases Risk for Dementia in Lewy Body Diseases http://www.lbda.org/content/genetic-mutation-increases-risk-dementia-lewy-body-diseases

[21] **Lennox G.** (2006) Managing Dementia and Parkinson's Disease. A PowerPoint presentation. http://www.bjhm.co.uk/ppts/(21-09-2006)parkinsons2006/managing-dementia-and-parkinsons-disease.ppt

[22] **Alzheimer's Association.** (2013) 2013 Alzheimer's Disease Facts and Figures, Alzheimer's & Dementia, Volume 9, Issue 2. http://www.alz.org/downloads/facts_figures_2013.pdf

[23] **Aarsland D, et al.** (2005) A systematic review of prevalence studies of dementia in Parkinson's disease. Mov Disord. 2005 Oct;20(10):1255-63. http://www.ncbi.nlm.nih.gov/pubmed/16041803

[24] **Susman E.** (2013) Mental Deficits Show Up Early in Parkinson's.17th Annual International Congress on Parkinson's Disease and Movement Disorders. MedPage Today, June 20, 2013. http://www.medpagetoday.com/MeetingCoverage/MDS/40000

[25] **Meireles J and Massano J.** (2012) Cognitive impairment and dementia in Parkinson's disease: clinical features, diagnosis, and management. Front. Neur. 3:88. doi: 10.3389/fneur.2012.00088. A review of the literature about these subjects through 2011. http://www.frontiersin.org/Dementia/10.3389/fneur.2012.00088/full

[26] **Aarsland D and Kurz MW.** (2010). The epidemiology of dementia associated with Parkinson disease. J. Neurol. Sci. 289, 18–22. doi: 10.1016/j.jns.2009.08.034. http://www.ncbi.nlm.nih.gov/pubmed/19733364

27 **Rana A, et al.** (2012) Prevalence and relation of dementia to various factors in Parkinson's disease. Psychiatry and Clinical Neurosciences 2012; 66: 64–68. http://onlinelibrary.wiley.com/doi/10.1111/j.1440-1819.2011.02291.x/pdf

28 **Remedy Health Media.** (2011) John Hopkins Health Alerts: Six Signs of Cognitive Impairment in Parkinson's Disease Patients. Sept 26, 2011. http://www.johnshopkinshealthalerts.com/alerts/memory/cognitive-impairment-Parkinsons_5902-1.html

29 **Parkinson's Disease Foundation.** (2013) Predicting Dementia in Early Parkinson's Disease. PDF, Science News. Apr 19, 2013. http://www.pdf.org/en/science_news/release/pr_1366397267

30 **Vyas U and Franco R.** (2012) REM Behavior Disorder (RBD) as an Early Marker for Development of Neurodegenerative Diseases. BJMP 2012;5(1):a506. http://www.bjmp.org/content/rem-behavior-disorder-rbd-early-marker-development-neurodegenerative-diseases

31 **Postuma R, et. al.** (2012) Rapid eye movement sleep behavior disorder and risk of dementia in Parkinson's disease: a prospective study. Movement Disorders, Volume 27, Issue 6, pages 720–726, May 2012. http://onlinelibrary.wiley.com/doi/10.1002/mds.24939/abstract

32 **Lane C.** (2014) General Depression. PsyWeb.com, Mon, December 01, 2014. http://www.psyweb.com/mdisord/jsp/gendepress.jsp

33 **Saczynski J S, et al.** (2010) Depressive symptoms and risk of dementia. Neurology July 6, 2010 vol. 75 no. 1 35-41. http://www.ncbi.nlm.nih.gov/pmc/articles/PMC2906404/

34 **Science Newsline, Medicine.** (2010) Mayo Clinic Study Finds Apathy And Depression Predict Progression from Mild Cognitive Impairment. Science Newsline, from **Geda Y E**, Mayo Clinic News, July 12, 2010. http://www.sciencenewsline.com/articles/2010071212000043.html

35 **Londos E, et al.** (2013) Dysphagia in Lewy body dementia - a clinical observational study of swallowing function by videofluoroscopic examination. BMC Neurology 2013, 13:140. http://www.biomedcentral.com/1471-2377/13/140

[36] **Susman E.** (2013) Docs Ignore Constipation in Parkinson's. 17th Annual International Congress on Parkinson's Disease and Movement Disorders. MedPage Today, June 17, 2013.
http://www.medpagetoday.com/MeetingCoverage/MDS/39901

[37] **Alzheimer's Society.** (2011) Urinary tract infection (UTI) and dementia. Fact Sheet 528. Reviewed 2011.
http://www.alzheimers.org.uk/site/scripts/documents_info.php?document ID=1777

[38] **Aarsland D, et al.** (2005) Neuroleptic sensitivity in Parkinson's disease and parkinsonian dementias. J Clin Psychiatry. 2005 May;66(5):633-7.
http://www.ncbi.nlm.nih.gov/pubmed/15889951

[39] **Pederson T.** (1997) The Unique Sensitivity of the Elderly. ExtoxNet FAQs on Sensitive Populations.
http://extoxnet.orst.edu/faqs/senspop/elder.htm

[40] **Drugs.com.** (2013) Benzodiazepines. http://www.drugs.com/drug-class/benzodiazepines.html

[41] **Billioti de GS** (2012) Benzodiazepine use and risk of dementia: prospective population based study BMJ 2012;345:e6231, 9-27-2012.
http://www.bmj.com/content/345/bmj.e6231

[42] **Collingwood J.** (2007). Inhaled Anesthetics Bring Alzheimer's Risk. Psych Central. http://psychcentral.com/lib/inhaled-anesthetics-bring-alzheimers-risk/000898

[43] **Pervin F and Lippa C.** (2014) Why Do Many People with LBD Respond Poorly to Surgery? Lewy Body Dementia Association, Ask the Expert. http://lbda.org/content/ask-expert-why-do-many-people-lbd-respond-poorly-surgery.

[44] **National Clinical Guideline Centre.** (2011) The Management of Hip Fracture in Adults. London: Royal College of Physicians (UK); 2011. NICE Clinical Guidelines, No. 124., 8, Regional (spinal or epidural) vs. general anesthesia. http://www.ncbi.nlm.nih.gov/books/NBK83023/

[45] **Barnett S, et. al.** (2009) Frequently Asked Questions About Anesthetic Considerations for Elderly Patients. American Society of Anesthesiologists Committee on Geriatric Anesthesia. http://www.sagahq.org/images/FAQs.pdf

[46] **Lewy Body Dementia Association.** (2008) LBD Medical Alert Wallet Card. http://lbda.org/content/lbd-medical-alert-wallet-card

[47] **Lewy Body Dementia Association.** (2012) Emergency Room Treatment of Psychosis. http://lbda.org/go/er

[48] **Leroi I, et. al.** (2011) Neuropsychiatric Symptoms in Parkinson's Disease with Mild Cognitive Impairment and Dementia. Parkinson's Disease, Volume 2012 (2012), Article ID 308097, 10 pages. http://www.hindawi.com/journals/pd/2012/308097/ref/

[49] **Munat F.** (2012) Be Brave. Unpublished book. http://florriemunat.com/contact_florrie_munat

[50] **Goetz CG, et al.** (2006). The malignant course of "benign" hallucinations in Parkinson's Disease. Archives of Neurology 63:713-716. http://www.ncbi.nlm.nih.gov/pubmed/16682540

[51] **eHealthMe.** (2012) Could Parkinson's disease cause Delusions? http://www.ehealthme.com/cs/parkinson's+disease/delusion

[52] **Phelps R and Leblanc G.** (2012) While I Still Can. Xlibris Corporation. http://whileistillcan.net/

[53] **Lewy Body Dementia Association.** (2010) Caregiver Burden in Lewy Body Dementia. http://lbda.org/go/caregiverburden

[54] **Manohor A and Galvin J.** (2011) Brain imaging for Lewy Body Dementia. Lewy Body Dementia Association, 3/16/2011. http://www.lbda.org/node/543

[55] **Alzheimer's Weekly.** (2013) Is It Lewy Body Dementia or Alzheimer's? Datscan Can Tell. Alzheimer's Weekly, March 24, 2013. http://www.alzheimersweekly.com/2013/03/is-it-lewy-body-dementia-or-alzheimers.html

[56] **Goldstein D.** (2012) Cardiac Sympathetic Neuroimaging in Dementia with Lewy Bodies. J Neuroimaging. 2012 April; 22(2): 109–110. http://www.ncbi.nlm.nih.gov/pmc/articles/PMC3030932/

[57] **Vertesi A, et al.** (2001) Standardized Mini-Mental State Examination. Use and interpretation. Canadian Family Physician, VOL 47: OCTOBER 2001 http://www.cfp.ca/content/47/10/2018.full.pdf

[58] **Palmqvist S, et al.** (2009) Practical suggestions on how to differentiate dementia with Lewy bodies from Alzheimer's disease with common cognitive tests. International Journal of Geriatric Psychiatry 2009; 24: 1405-1412. http://www.ncbi.nlm.nih.gov/pubmed/19347836

[59] **Carolan Doerflinger D.** (2012) Mental Status Assessment in Older Adults: Montreal Cognitive Assessment: MoCA Version 7.1 (Original Version) From a 2012 Series provided by the Hartford Institute of Geriatric Nursing, NYU, College of Nursing. http://consultgerirn.org/uploads/File/trythis/try_this_3_2.pdf

[60] **Changing Minds.org** (2002-2012) The Kübler-Ross Grief Cycle. Disciplines, Change Management. http://changingminds.org/disciplines/change_management/kubler_ross/kubler_ross.htm

[61] **Jennings J.** (2012) Living with Lewy Body Dementia. One Caregiver's Personal In-depth Experience. (2012) WestBow Press. Blog: http://www.ourlewybodydementiaadventure.com/ Book: http://www.lbdtools.com/shop_books.html

[62] **Meyyappan R.** (2013) LBD and Social Security Disability Benefits. The Lewy Body Rollercoaster, June 8, 2013 blog. http://lewybodydementia.blogspot.com/2013/06/lbd-and-social-security-disability.html

[63] **Jong N.** (2013) Activities of Daily Living (ADLs) SeniorHomes.com. http://www.seniorhomes.com/p/activities-of-daily-living/

[64] **Marak C.** (2015) Activities of Daily Living (ADLs) Assisted living serves those that need assistance with ADLs. AssistedLivingFacilities.org. 2015. http://www.assistedlivingfacilities.org/resources/services-provided/activities-of-daily-living-adls-/

[65] **Medicaid.gov.**(2013) Spousal Impoverishment.
http://medicaid.gov/Medicaid-CHIP-Program-Information/By-Topics/Eligibility/Spousal-Impoverishment-Page.html

[66] **U.S. Department of Veterans Affairs**. (2013) Guide to Long Term Care. Geriatrics and Extended Care.
http://www.va.gov/GERIATRICS/Guide/LongTermCare/index.asp

[67] **Despues D.** (1999) Stress and Illness. California State University, Northridge. Spring, 1999.
http://www.csun.edu/~vcpsy00h/students/illness.htm

[68] **Changing Minds.** (2002) (Fight-or-Flight Reaction. Changing Minds.org. (2002-2015)
http://changingminds.org/explanations/brain/fight_flight.htm

[69] **Collingwood J.** (2007) The Physical Effects of Long-Term Stress. PsychCentral. http://psychcentral.com/lib/the-physical-effects-of-long-term-stress/000935?all=1

[70] **Memory People Facebook Page**. A closed group for dementia victims, their caregivers and advocates.

[71] **Olpin M.** (2010) The World is NOT a Stressful Place, Eloquent Books, 2010. Chapter 13.
http://faculty.weber.edu/molpin/healthclasses/1110/bookchapters/musicchapter.htm

[72] **Armstrong RA.** (2011) Visual Symptoms in Parkinson's Disease. Parkinson's Disease. Volume 2011, Article ID 908306. Hindawi Publishing Corp. http://www.hindawi.com/journals/pd/2011/908306/

[73] **Ramig L, et al.** (2009) The Science and Practice of "Speaking LOUD" and "Moving BIG." 2009, APDA, Midwest Chapter.
http://www.apdamidwest.org/APDA_Midwest/Speaking_LOUD.html

[74] **BrightFocus Foundation** (2014) Alzheimer's Prevention & Risk Factors. About Alzheimer's. March, 2014.
http://www.brightfocus.org/alzheimers/about/risk/

[75] **Lourinda I, et al.** (2013) Mediterranean Diet, Cognitive Function, and Dementia: A Systematic Review.
http://www.ncbi.nlm.nih.gov/pubmed/23680940

[76] **Cassels C** (2013) Novel Exercise Program May Trump Meds for Dementia. Medscape Today, Mar 28, 2013. http://www.medscape.com/viewarticle/781607

[77] **Ryan** (2012) Four Scientific Findings that point to the importance of Brain Fitness for the Aging Population brain. 5/29/2012. http://www.marblesthebrainstore.com/files/Brain_Fitness_for_the_Aging_Population.pdf

[78] **Aubrey A.** (2010) Mental Stimulation Postpones, Then Speeds Dementia. NPR News. September 4, 2010 http://www.npr.org/templates/story/story.php?storyId=129628082

[79] **Jennings J.** (2012) (See Reference #61)

[80] **Levine B.** (2011) Warding Off Dementia. Baseline of Health Foundation Health Blog. 6/21/2011. http://www.jonbarron.org/article/warding-dementia

[81] **Ramig L, et al.** (2009) (See Reference #73)

[82] **JeanneG** (2012) Fore! LBDA forum, LBD Clinical Issues, Treatment Options. June 9, 2012. http://community.lbda.org/forum/viewtopic.php?f=4&t=3483

[83] **Schneider C.** (2006) Don't Bury Me…It Ain't Over Yet. Author House. http://www.lbdtools.com/shop_books.html

[84] **Jennings J.** (2012) (See Reference # 61)

[85] **Silver H.** (2009) "Food Modification versus Oral Liquid Nutrition Supplementation." The Economic, Medical/Scientific and Regulatory Aspects of Clinical Nutrition Practice: What Impacts What? Ed. M Elia and B Bistrian. Nestec Ltd, 2009.Vol 12, pp 79-93. Web. 5 Mar. 2013. Accessed 3/5/13: http://www.nestlenutrition-institute.org/resources/library/Free/workshop/BookNNIW12/Documents/NNW012079.pdf

[86] **Jones P.** (2008) Sleeping Aids for Seniors and Seniors With Dementia: Melatonin and Zolpidem. Beth Israel Deaconess Medical Center. July, 2008. http://www.bidmc.org/YourHealth/Health-Research-Journals.aspx?ChunkID=330428

[87] **Tsuang D, et al.** (2010) Association between lifetime cigarette smoking and Lewy body accumulation. Brain Pathol. 2010 March; 20(2): 412–18. http://www.ncbi.nlm.nih.gov/pmc/articles/PMC2864364/

[88] **Tubeza P.** (2013) FDA warns on dangers of e-cigarettes. Philippine Daily Inquirer, June 27, 2013. http://newsinfo.inquirer.net/434233/fda-warns-on-dangers-of-e-cigarettes

[89] **Boston University Medical Center** (2010) Moderate drinking, especially wine, associated with better cognitive function. ScienceDaily, 08/2010. http://www.sciencedaily.com/releases/2010/08/100818085651.htm

[90] **Dartmouth College, Academic Skills Center.** (2006) Alcohol and Sleep. Academic Skills Center, Dartmouth College 2001 BASICS – A Harm Reduction Approach. Oregon State University. http://studenthealth.oregonstate.edu/sites/default/files/docs/alcohol_and_sleep.pdf

[91] **Healy M.** (2015) Marijuana pills fail to ease dementia symptoms. Los Angeles Times, May 13, 2015.http://www.latimes.com/science/sciencenow/la-sci-sn-marijuana-pill-dementia-20150513-story.html

[92] **Sharma P.** (2012) Chemistry, Metabolism, and Toxicology of Cannabis: Clinical Implications. Iran J Psychiatry. 2012 Fall; 7(4): 149–156.http://www.ncbi.nlm.nih.gov/pmc/articles/PMC3570572/

[93] **Jaffee S.** (2013) Therapy Plateau No Longer Ends. The New Old Age. Caring and Coping. http://newoldage.blogs.nytimes.com/2013/02/04/therapy-plateau-no-longer-ends-coverage/?hp

[94] **Snyder P.** (2012) Treasures in the Darkness. CreateSpace Independent Publishing. http://www.lbdtools.com_store.html

[95] **Simons-Stern N, et al.** (2010) Music as a Memory Enhancer in Patients with Alzheimer's Disease. Neuropsychologia. 2010 Aug; 48(10): 3164–3167. http://www.ncbi.nlm.nih.gov/pmc/articles/PMC2914108/

[96] **Pacchetti C, et al.** (2000) Active music therapy in Parkinson's disease: an integrative method for motor and emotional rehabilitation. Psychosom

Med. 2000 May-Jun;62(3):386-93.
http://www.ncbi.nlm.nih.gov/pubmed/10845352

[97] **University of California - Davis** (2009) Brain Hub That Links Music, Memory And Emotion Discovered. ScienceDaily, February 24, 2009. http://www.sciencedaily.com/releases/2009/02/090223221230.htm

[98] **Omar R, et al.** (2011) The structural neuroanatomy of music emotion recognition: Evidence from frontotemporal lobar degeneration. NCBI.Neuroimage. 2011 June 1; 56(3): 1814–1821. http://www.ncbi.nlm.nih.gov/pmc/articles/PMC3092986/

[99] **Snyder P.** (See Reference #94)

[100] **Bucznski R.** (2012) Does Spirituality Belong in Therapy. National Institute for the Clinical Application of Behavioral Medicine. July 25, 2012. http://www.nicabm.com/nicabmblog/spirituality-in-therapy

[101] **Fung J, et. al.** (2012) A systematic review of the use of aromatherapy in treatment of behavioral problems in dementia. Geriatrics & Geriatr Gerontol Int 2012; 12: 372–382.20 http://onlinelibrary.wiley.com/doi/10.1111/j.1447-0594.2012.00849.x/abstract

[102] **Lanza S.** (2007) Aromatherapy in Dementia Care. The Dementia Caregiver's Toolbox, Parts 1, 2 and 3. November 18, 20 and 23, 2007. http://nurturingnuggets.typepad.com/the_nurturing_nuggets_blo/2007/11/aromatherapy-in.html

[103] **Robbins W.** (2015) Aromatherapy and Anosmia (Loss of the Sense of Smell). AromaWeb. http://www.aromaweb.com/articles/aromatherapy-anosmia-loss-sense-of-smell.asp

[104] **Stone A.** (2014) Smell Turns Up in Unexpected Places. The New York Times, Oct. 13, 2014. http://www.nytimes.com/2014/10/14/science/smell-turns-up-in-unexpected-places.html?_r=1

[105] **Baldauf M P.** (2011, Dec 27) "In Memory Of My Father, Richard Baldauf." Every Woman Blog. Posted on http://everywomanblog.com/2011/12/

[106] **British Acupuncture Council** (2013) Dementia. Back to Research Fact Sheet. March 28, 2013. http://www.acupuncture.org.uk/a-to-z-of-conditions/a-to-z-of-conditions/3202-dementia.html

[107] **Yang M-H**, et al. (2007) The efficacy of acupressure for decreasing agitated behavior in dementia: a pilot study. J Clin Nurs. 2007 Feb;16(2):308-15. http://www.ncbi.nlm.nih.gov/pubmed/17239066

[108] **British Acupuncture Council** (2013) Dementia. Back to Research Fact Sheet. March 28, 2013. http://www.acupuncture.org.uk/a-to-z-of-conditions/a-to-z-of-conditions/3202-dementia.html

[109] **Yang M-H**, et al. (2007) The efficacy of acupressure for decreasing agitated behavior in dementia: a pilot study. J Clin Nurs. 2007 Feb;16(2):308-15. http://www.ncbi.nlm.nih.gov/pubmed/17239066

[110] **Viggo H N**,et al. (2006) Massage and touch for dementia. Cochrane Database Syst Rev. 2006 Oct 18;(4):CD004989. http://www.ncbi.nlm.nih.gov/pubmed/17054228

[111] **Lewy Body Dementia Association.** (2007) Research Shows LBD Places High Toll on Families. 12/31/2007. http://lbda.org/node/194

[112] **Boström F.** (2007) Patients with Lewy body dementia use more resources than those with Alzheimer's disease. Int J Geriatr Psychiatry. 2007 Aug;22(8):713-9. http://www.ncbi.nlm.nih.gov/pubmed/17195278

[113] **Fereshtehnejad S-M.** (2014) Co-morbidity profile in DLB vs. AD: a linkage study between the Swedish Dementia Registry and the Swedish National Patient Registry. Alzheimer's Research & Therapy 2014, 6:65. http://alzres.com/content/6/5/65

[114] **Galvin J.** (2010) LBD-Caregiver burden in Lewy Body Dementias. Alzheimer Dis Assoc Disord. 2010 Apr-Jun;24(2):177-81. Lewy Body Dementia Association. http://lbda.org/node/295

[115] **Snyder P.** (See Reference # 94)

[116] **Scarff S and Zultner A.** (2012) Dementia. The Journey Ahead. Langdon Street Press, MN. Blog: http://www.dementiathejourneyahead.com/ Book: http://www.lbdtools.com/shop_books.html

[117] **Walker J.** (2011) Three Years and Thirteen Dumpsters: Cleaning House After Dementia. CreateSpace Independent Publishing.
Blog: http://cleaninghousebook.blogspot.com/
Book: www.lbdtools.com/shop_books.html

[118] **Schneider C.** (See Reference # 83)

[119] **Wesolowski K.** (2010) When Should People With Dementia Stop Driving? Neurology Now: May/June 2010 - Volume 6 - Issue 3 - p 11
http://journals.lww.com/neurologynow/Fulltext/2010/06030/When_Should_People_With_Dementia_Stop_Driving_.8.aspx

[120] **CaregiverStress.com.** (2010) The 50/50 Rule: Solving Family Conflict.
http://www.caregiverstress.com/family-communication/solving-family-conflict/sharing-care-plans/

[121] **Carriere I** (2009) Drugs with anticholinergic properties, cognitive decline, and dementia in an elderly general population: the 3-city study. Arch Intern Med. 2009 Jul; 169(14): 1317–1324.
http://www.ncbi.nlm.nih.gov/pmc/articles/PMC2933398/

[122] **Scarff S and Zultner A.** (See Reference # 114)

[123] **Agingcare.com.** Obsessive Compulsive Disorder (OCD) in Elders. National Institutes of Health.
http://www.agingcare.com/Articles/obsessive-compulsive-disorder-in-elderly-parents-138686.htm

[124] **Parkinson's Disease Foundation.** (2010) The Ups and Downs of Dopamine: Impulse Control and Parkinson's. An Interview with Dr. Daniel Weintraub. News and Review.
http://www.pdf.org/pdf/NL_Fall_10.pdf

[125] **Snyder Pat.** (See Reference #94)

[126] **Whitworth, H.** (2013) Hospice is for Life not Death. The Lewy Body Rollercoaster. blog, June 15, 2013.
http://lewybodydementia.blogspot.com/2013/06/hospice-is-for-life-not-death.html

69027160R00193

Made in the USA
Lexington, KY
24 October 2017